Acting Healthy

*"If all the world's a stage, how do we play a
bigger part in our own lives?"*

MARY MILLER

Acting Healthy

Directors Notes for a Better Life

Mary Miller

ACTING HEALTHY is a new take on wellness using acting tips and techniques to help you play a bigger, happier, thinner, younger, healthier part in your own life! After all the first step to being happy, thin, young, and healthy is acting happy, thin, young, and healthy every day.

Directors Notes for a Better Life are daily insights into theatre and life that will help you begin to make a change. In theatre director's notes are those notes given to actors after a rehearsal to help make a better play. Why not use them here to help make a better life?

ACTING HEALTHY: Directors Notes for a Better Life is a daily journal. A mixture of theatre and self-help designed to entertain as well as give you the acting tools you need to make a difference in your life. Each day starts with a new thought ... that thought is explored ... and then brought to life by an excerpt from a play.

MARY MILLER

INTRODUCTION

I read where a schoolboy once wrote that Socrates used to go around giving advice so they poisoned him! So, I'm well aware of the danger of giving advice. But I have been writing plays that have changed people's lives for years. I have watched the effect of what I have written move an audience to laughter and tears. I have won awards for every play I have written. I've seen my work produced across the United States and around the world. I know the research and care that went into writing each story. I know that theatre can change your life. My goal is to help people understand they do have a choice and theatre can lead the way!

LIGHTS! CAMERA!! ACTION!!!
Mary Miller

For more information: _www.actinghealthy.com_

MARY MILLER

January 1st

Want a better life? Write a better play!

If all the world is a stage ... how do we play a bigger part in our own lives? Why not write a better role? Think about it. The mind and body connection is a theatrical event. It's theatre at its best! We are the actors in our own lives. If we choose to be happy we can be happy. If we choose to be sad we can be sad. If we choose to be thin ... we can be thin! We can write the play we want to play and act the part we want to be. Who better to tell you how, than a playwright?

CLARICE: You can do it now.

BERNICE: I haven't acted in years.

CLARICE: Hush! You acted every day of your life when you went into Sunshine and Sholtz and "acted" like a secretary.

Excerpt from the play <u>Mulberry Lane</u> by Mary Miller

January 2nd

Why me?

First it is important to know the plays I write focus on the human condition – our fears, our joys, our pains, our sorrows, our hopes, our dreams, and our *health*. It's the human condition that fascinates me. I don't write high-action-dramas like the *Bourne Identity* – where Matt Damon wakes up, doesn't know who he is, and finds out that the CIA is chasing him! That's a wonderful story and I wish I had written it! But the story that interests me is not waking up and *not knowing* who you are but waking up and *knowing* exactly who you are and what you have to do to get through the day. Sometimes the greatest conflict in life can be simply getting out of bed and putting one foot in front of the other!

JOHN: Excuse me. Excuse me? I hope I'm not ... crowding you ...

DORIE: (flustered/embarrassed) No.

(He slides into the empty seat and sits next to her.)

Excerpt from the play <u>Ferris Wheel</u> by Mary Miller

January 3rd

Why you?

Now let me ask you a question. First, what play are you living? Is it a drama, comedy, soap opera, sitcom, tragedy, farce or a long running saga? Do you want to continue living in that genre? Second, if they had a casting call to play the part of your life would you audition for the role? Would you take it if you got it? If the answer to any of these questions is "no" or even a half-hearted "maybe" then Acting Healthy is for you! LIGHTS. CAMERA. ACTION.

DORIE: Whoops...we're off!!

Excerpt from the play Ferris Wheel by Mary Miller

January 4th

Finding Your Part

People tell me, this idea of Acting Healthy is OK for you, you have an imagination, you've created characters in your mind and written them down on paper and acted them out on stage. But what about me? How do I begin to know what character I want to play? It's easier than you think. The beauty of acting is you don't have to be yourself. The quickest way to find the part you want to play is by copying a character you already like. Think of a character … any character. From the movies or TV or someone at work. Make a choice and then for 24 hours act like that character. You don't have to tell anyone what you are doing … in fact it's best not to! See if acting like someone else doesn't give you some insight into how you want to act in your own life.

MASON: (surprised) You are jealous.

L.E.: (defensive) Of Merrillee?! I most certainly am not. Why would I be jealous of her?

Excerpt from the play Light Burgers by Mary Miller

January 5th

Writing the Dialogue

All great plays, including yours, begin with the word. The word is what we tell ourselves, over and over, day after day, usually without any thought. It's our *internal* dialogue. "I'm fat. I'm ugly. I'm sick. I'm tired. I'm old." Sound familiar? We are what we say we are. But what are we saying? And is that really what we mean? Probably not. But we've grown so accustomed to hearing it I doubt we realize that we are the ones perpetuating it. The first thing we have to do to change our life is to change our dialogue ... both internal and external. To change your dialogue you don't have to buy any fancy equipment. You don't have to write morning, noon, and night! You don't even have to spend any money. You just have to change how you think! The quickest way to change how you think is to change how you act! Whether it's acting happy, acting thin, acting young, or acting healthy!

CLARICE: First we have to get you a resume!

BERNICE: A resume?! I haven't done anything ...

CLARICE: Oh, hush. You have too — we'll make it up. Where's your pen. (She takes Bernice's pen and writes on the flyer.) 99% of all the resumes on Broadway were made up at some time.

Excerpt from the play Mulberry Lane by Mary Miller

January 6th

Acting Thin

What if losing weight could be as easy as acting thin? It's possible. Try this. Next time you sit down to a meal instead of looking at the food and saying *"I'm going to gain weight"* try saying *"I'm going to lose weight."* You're going to eat it anyway, right? What's the difference, you ask? Ah!! The difference is you changed your dialogue and in doing so you changed your mind. When you change your mind you change how you act. Suddenly it's not a sin to eat it anymore. Suddenly it's not the thrill it was a minute before. Suddenly you have more power over what you are eating. Suddenly you give yourself permission to lose weight.

ALLISON: In an hour you'd be hungry again?

LOUISE: In an hour I'll be hungry again anyway.

Excerpt from the play Waiting for Oprah by Mary Miller

January 7th

Acting Thin: Accentuate the Positive

Did you know that the brain cannot process a negative? When you see a *"Do Not Touch"* sign what's the first thing you want to do? Touch it! Right? It's the same with food. You hear *"Don't eat that!"* and the first thing you want to do is *eat it!* (No matter what it is?!) You are powerless. You can't stop thinking about it. You think about it all day. You think about it during lunch. You think about it during dinner. It'll pop into your head in the middle of the night! It will drive you crazy! The reason? What you say and what your brain actually hears are two different things! You say *"don't eat that"* but the brain hears *"eat that."* By the time you've reprocessed the thought, backtracked it in your mind, and reinterpreted *"eat that"* back to *"**don't** eat that,"* nine times out of ten you've already eaten it! Change your dialogue and change your mind. Accentuate the positive and take your power back.

JANICE: At least I tried.

ALLISON: You did at that ... and the table was lovely.

JANICE: It was, wasn't it?

LOUISE: It wasn't your fault everyone got drunk.

ALLISON: They just couldn't eat the food.

Excerpt from the play <u>Waiting for Oprah</u> by Mary Miller

January 8th

Acting Thin: Directing the Action

Why is it when we eat a wonderful meal somewhere during the process someone will always say: "This is delicious but it's going straight to my hip ... my thighs ... my stomach!" You've heard it before. You may have even said it yourself. Stop it! Because the only thing you are doing when you say things like this is directing the food to go to your hips, your thighs, your stomach! Honestly. Our bodies do exactly what we tell them to do. Stop directing your food to go to places you don't want. Enjoy what you eat and say no more!

BABS: Look Momma. There's coleslaw, mashed potatoes, biscuits and gravy. That's Christmassy?

LIZBETH: Even plastic forks and knives and paper plates. All the conveniences of home.

MARGARET: And eggnog! One day we'll look back on this and laugh.

Excerpt from the play <u>A Christmas House</u> by Mary Miller

January 9th

Acting Thin: Look at me!

When you eat look at your food. Smile at it. Literally!! Look at it and smile. So often we eat without looking we're surprised when we're finished! It may sound strange but the more you enjoy your food, really enjoy it, indulge in it, savor it while you are eating it the better your health and digestion will be. Smile at your food … give yourself permission to eat what you want … but the moment you stop looking at your food stop eating. It's as simple as that. You don't have to eat the whole pie to enjoy one bite.

LOUISE: I can't believe I ate that whole display!

JANICE: It was much more appetizing than those gummy-worms Mia had hanging all over everything when we were reading that book about The Plague.

Excerpt from the play <u>Waiting for Oprah</u> by Mary Miller

January 10th

Acting Thin: A Real Sense of Loss

One of the things they don't tell you when you lose weight is that there can be a real sense of pain. A sense of loss. A personal loss as if someone had died. In fact part of you will die. The part of you who eats with you. The part of you who tells you it's OK, you deserve it. The part of you who allows you to comfort yourself with food. Losing weight can feel like losing a lover, a companion, a friend. When someone loses 100 pounds it's the equivalent to losing a person! No one ever talks about weight loss in terms of personal loss. I believe that's why so many diets don't work, because when you get down to the nitty-gritty you miss that part of yourself and it's frightening. It's downright scary. It's like going on stage alone. The spotlight hits you and you have no one to turn to but yourself and you don't know who you are. You don't know what to say. You don't know how to act. At least not yet.

CHILD: I don't know how to talk to other people.

WOMAN: You just open up your mouth and say "Hello!". People will talk to you. Talk to you more than you want to hear, if you let 'em.

CHILD: They won't be you.

WOMAN: Well, you got such a powerful memory you just think back to some of those hours we had and they'll keep you company, 'til something better comes along. You hear?

Excerpt from the play Take Proper Care by Mary Miller

January 11th

Acting Happy: The Real Fountain Of Youth!

Some days it seems we've gotten so sophisticated we've sophisticated ourselves out of our own happiness! Being happy in my opinion stops the aging process, enlivens the spirit, lifts the heart, and gives us all a reason to live! When we're happy we never ask the question *"why are we here?"* The answer is clear. We're here to enjoy life, enjoy nature, enjoy each other, and enjoy ourselves! Want to attract happiness in your life? The first step is to smile.

L.E.: Will you stop it! Nothing is going to happen! No UFO is going to land here!

MASON: I wish it would.

MERRILLEE: That's the first step in attracting a UFO, Mason, is just wishing it would come...thinking pleasant thoughts, non-threatening things like: I want you to come. I believe you are coming. You're so pretty, I wish you would come closer. We all respond to pleasant things after all it's only human.

Excerpt from the play <u>Light Burgers</u> by Mary Miller

January 12th

Acting Happy: Casting

Have you ever noticed when you're having a good day nothing can bring you down? When you're having a bad day everything brings you down. It's like you attract bad luck. I believe it's true. You do! You attract the emotions you put out. Good or bad. Happy or sad. It's the same with people too. Happy people attract happy people. So, when you're casting your life with the characters you want around you, look for happy people to populate your stage. They're not hard to find. They're the ones smiling!!

MASON: Personally, I don't see anything wrong with having something out there that you can't explain. I find it comforting. And if I do say so myself, you are looking particularly nice this evening Merrillee.

MERRILLEE: (smiling) Why, thank you Mason. My Mamma used to say it's always important to look your best. After all, you never get a second chance to make a good first impression ... no matter where you're going.

Excerpt from the play Light Burgers by Mary Miller

January 13th

Acting Happy: Unhappy Past

One of the things that cause us to miss our own happiness is our tendency to focus on the past. Of course, the older we get the more past we have and whether we like it or not, feelings and emotions get tangled up in our brain. We find ourselves living in the past – literally. The smallest thing can trigger it. Focus on a bad memory 20 years ago and you will feel it as if it were happening again now. If you continue to re-play that memory you will eventually hardwire your brain for pain. So to be happy you have to let that memory go. You don't have to forget it; you just have to stop reliving it day after day.

JACKSON: I can't take any more from you Momma. I won't.

(She looks at the money in her hand and puts it back in her robe. She looks up at Jackson and takes his face in her hands.)

PEARL: I spec you can't. It's just I see so much of your Daddy in you 'til it near 'bout breaks my heart. You do what you have to do and don't you pay no 'tention to what this old woman says.

Excerpt from the play I Witness by Mary Miller

13

January 14ᵗʰ

Acting Happy: Make a New Memory

If you find yourself saddened by the past, stop thinking about the past, change your mind, think of something else, get up and walk around the room. Did you know that it's virtually impossible to stay in a negative mindset if you are moving! So if you find yourself rolled up in a ball underneath the covers in your bed (reading this entry!) get up, get dressed, get going, and make a new memory. A better memory. A happy memory!

MATTIE: Chandler!! You made it! You should have called! (hugging her) I can't believe it's you. I was afraid you wouldn't come.

CHANDLER: I couldn't very well ignore a telegram saying: "STOP! Virgin crying in our backyard!!"

Excerpt from the play <u>Virgin Tears</u> by Mary Miller

January 15th

Acting Happy: Method Acting vs. Being

When I first went to New York I studied *Method Acting*. The process involved getting on stage and remembering a moment in life and reliving it. Most people used the *Method* to get to tears. Think of a miserable time where you cried, relive that moment, and cry again! The audience won't know why you are crying, they'll just see real tears, and you can get a job on a soap opera! The problem with the *Method* is it doesn't last ... not with tears ... not with laughter (and people can tell the difference!) Years later I studied with Mira Rostova who literately helped me *become* the character. She helped me learn how to believe I was the character I was playing on stage whether I was happy or sad and my emotions flowed. That's what I'm talking about. Being the part. It's not just being an actor on stage, it's becoming the person you want to be in life.

BERNICE: Don't you tell me what I should or shouldn't have done. I'm far too old and there's too much water under the bridge to worry about a stupid old dream.

CLARICE: You could do it now!

Excerpt from the play <u>Mulberry Lane</u> by Mary Miller

January 16ᵗʰ

Acting Happy: Make Someone Happy

The best tip I can give you on how to be happy and stay happy is to open yourself up to other people. Change your internal dialogue from what someone can do to make you happy to what you can do to make someone else happy. I am not talking about buying them *stuff*. We are so conditioned to believe that *stuff* will make us happy and it doesn't. Oh, it might for the moment, but not forever. And when it falls short we are even more unhappy. Instead of *"make my day"* ... make someone else's day. Happiness is a muscle ... exercise it. Strengthen it. Have the courage to be happy. It's OK, you don't have to feel guilty for all the unhappy people in the world; your being depressed won't help them at all. You don't have to worry about the other shoe falling! Everyone is entitled to be happy.

MATTIE: Then you'll help me?

CHANDLER: Bore a hole?

MATTIE: No! Eye-drop a tear. Please, Chandler. Just one little tear. It wouldn't be hard and it'd mean the world to Adele. I'd do it myself, but I can't. I've tried ... three times ... but every time I got close to the Virgin my hands shook so hard I didn't think they'd ever stop. That's when I decided to call you. I thought you, of all the people I knew, could do it and then the Virgin would cry for us all.

Excerpt from the play <u>Virgin Tears</u> by Mary Miller

January 17th

Acting Young

The truth is youth is all about enthusiasm. Young and old alike. Have you ever met a young person who seemed old? Now I don't want to be a teenager again. I've been there, done that! But I also don't want to pick up the cloak of old-age and drape it over my shoulders. The problem is we set benchmarks in our mind as we age: 30, 40, 50, 60, and so on. In doing so we set ourselves up to age whether we mean to or not. After all what we've set up in our minds … we create in our bodies. Folks will argue with me and say at _____ (you fill in the age) the body starts to fall apart, but who's to say we didn't put that thought into our head 20 years ago? Before our body actually started to fall apart! And now we're living that image? We say as we age our metabolism slows down. We say our eyes give out. We say we can't do what we did as a young person. Maybe so … maybe not. Maybe we can do more? Ask yourself – how old you would be if you didn't know how old you were? Now act that way.

MARGARET: The other day I found myself standing in line, signing up for one of those single matchmaking type groups.

LIZBETH: I think that's great.

MARGARET: Except I lied on my application card. The group is supposed to be under 30. So, I fudged a bit on my age. Why do they make such a big deal over age? It's all in your mind anyway.

BABS: And how old are you … in your mind?

Excerpt from the play <u>A Christmas House</u> by Mary Miller

January 18th

Acting Young: Lie about your age!

For six years in New York City I was 22 years old. I figured 22 was the optimum age to be an actor in New York ... so for six years I said I was 22. The interesting thing is while I was pretending to be 22, I felt 22, I acted like I was 22, I experienced life like I was 22, I got cast as a 22 year old and I believe for those six years I didn't experience aging the same way I might have otherwise. Somehow during the time I was pretending to be 22, I didn't age the same way as the rest of my friends ... who were aging one year older every year. I can't prove it but I believe it. Einstein has a theory about this called the *Twin Paradox Theory*. Einstein believed that if you took two identical twins and sent one off into deep space while the other one remained at home on Earth the space traveling twin when he returned would be younger than his home bound brother! So, if we can experience time differently from Einstein's point of view ... who's to say we can't experience time differently in our own life ... without having to take a trip into deep space ... maybe we can experience time differently by just lying about our age.

CLARICE: I wouldn't say so if I didn't. And have you ever known me to lie?

BERNICE: About your age, your weight, your hair color, your...

CLARICE: About something important?

BERNICE: (giving in) No.

Excerpt from the play <u>Mulberry Lane</u> by Mary Miller

January 19th

Acting Young: Do something you love.

Do what you love. It's not a new thought. But it is a true thought. You don't have to make a living doing it, in fact it's probably better not to try, but the path to real happiness and true youth is to do something you love at least once a day … everyday. Why? Because doing something you love will remind you that you're alive. Sometimes we get so caught up in the pressures of the world and the constant rushing from here to there that we forget how to live the life we imagined when we were kids. People say the difference between old-age and youth is that the young believe we can solve the problems of the world and old-age knows we can't. But what if we could? To stay young do something you love … you'll never be as young as you are in this moment!

BABS: I thought you were doing what you wanted to do.

MARGARET: I'm doing what I thought I should be doing.

LIZBETH: What do you want to do?

MARGARET: I don't know. That's the problem. I've always done what other people wanted me to do. I've never really thought much about what I wanted to do, until now, and I'm still not sure … but straight hair is a start!

Excerpt from the play <u>A Christmas House</u> by Mary Miller

January 20th

Acting Healthy: To be or not to be.

In this world of realism it seems we are all predisposed to talk of our health in terms of illness rather than wellness. It's a part of the vernacular. For some reason it sounds more *realistic* to be sick rather than to be healthy. I believe our body will do whatever you ask of it. So don't ask for illnesses when the goal is wellness. Don't say I get a cold every winter unless you want one. Don't say you feel sick unless you are sick. Even the sentence "I never get sick" sends the wrong message to your brain. It trips you up. I've talked about the fact that the brain doesn't understand the concept of a negative and nowhere else does this come into play more than talking about health. This doesn't mean you should ignore an illness or avoid check ups. I just mean when given a choice act healthy.

FRAN: Eventually we will all die.

JANICE: Hypothetically.

ALLISON: Hypothetically my foot! It's a fact: Death and Taxes.

LOUISE: No need in speeding it up today.

Excerpt from the play <u>Waiting for Oprah</u> by Mary Miller

January 21st

Acting Healthy: A Time To Change

Change is not something we like to accept, but change happens. There are two major changes that occur when we get older: changes in our body and changes around us. Changes in our body we equate most often with disease. Changes around us can be something as detached as a building being built or torn down or as personal as losing a job or a loved one. The landscape around us changes, for better or worse, and it's unsettling both inside and out! No one can escape change. The question is how you handle it and how you handle it can change your life. Start by distinguishing what you can and cannot change and embrace the difference. Don't be afraid. *The Times They Are A Changing* is a song Bob Dylan wrote in 1963 ... the times they were a changing then and they are still changing now. At a faster clip than we ever imagined!

CHILD: I don't know how I'm going to live without you.

WOMAN: You'll start back to school in a couple days, and you'll be so busy you won't have time to think about me.

CHILD: I hate things to change.

WOMAN: Change ain't always bad. It ain't ever easy. But it ain't always bad.

Excerpt from the play Take Proper Care by Mary Miller

January 22nd

Acting Healthy: A New Normal

On Tuesday June 6, 2000, I was diagnosed with Endometrial cancer and by that Friday night I had a radical hysterectomy. Change happens. It can happen fast. I wasn't feeling bad. In fact, I couldn't have been in better health … except for this cancer growing in my uterus! Talk about being thrown for a loop. My book *A Christmas House* (originally titled *Unfinished Dreams*) had just come out. I did a book signing the Saturday before I got the diagnosis and I had my entire life planned … except for this! It felt strange then, it feels strange now. Suddenly I was faced with what would ultimately become a "new normal" for me. Now on every health form that bit of information has to be listed. Every check-up is checked with a little more scrutiny. For the next five years my life went on hold until I got the all clear sign. That five-year marker that says you're cured and you can now go on with the rest of your life. Life is like that, full of fits and starts. It's not how you stop that matters … it's how you start again that determines your life. Change happens. And it's OK.

LOUISE: And you're sure …

FRAN: I'm sure.

ALLISON: You talked to a doctor?

FRAN: Not at first. At first, he wouldn't go to a doctor. He's a grown man, it's not like a child you can pick up and take. He knew he was having problems long before I realized it … I was willing to let it slide we all forget things periodically.

Excerpt from the play <u>Waiting for Oprah</u> by Mary Miller

January 23rd

Act Now

Love is the most overused expression in the English language ... if you ask me. Love is used to buy and sell everything. We do anything for love. But what does it mean: to love? The romantics will tell you it's of the heart. The optimistic will say it's all around you. The pessimists will say it just passed you by. Love is not a Hallmark card. It's not cupid. It's not Valentine's Day ... although many industries depend on it. Love is what you feel inside for another person, place, or thing that elevates it above the rest. Love can be fleeting or long lasting. Joyful or painful. Love may be all around you but where it lives is in your mind. Think love ... and act on it now.

BERNICE (totally frustrated): Clarice, I didn't love George! I didn't want to marry George!

CLARICE: What do you mean you didn't love George? He was the only person I ever knew who could make you babble like a schoolgirl.

Excerpt from the play <u>Mulberry Lane</u> by Mary Miller

January 24th

Act Now: 30 - 30 - 30 School for Actors

How do you build a relationship? It starts with the willingness to connect with people on a real personal level. The quickest way to do that is what I call my *30-30-30 School for Actors*. 30 Seconds. 30 Minutes. 30 Days. Here's how it works! *30 SECONDS:* Within the first 30 seconds of a conversation with anyone say something encouraging or complimentary. The trick here is it has to be something genuine, specific, and real. In other words it has to be true! *30 MINUTES:* For 30 minutes each day think of what you have to be grateful for. Think about what you love. It can be simple or complex but give yourself at least 30 minutes a day. The key here is that it doesn't have to be 30 minutes in a row! But it should add up to 30 minutes in a day!! *30 DAYS:* For the next 30 days stand in front of a mirror and say "I love you." Say it out loud and say it as if you really mean it! That's the acting part! See if by the end of the month you haven't fallen in love with yourself and maybe, just maybe, someone will have fallen in love with you! 30 seconds. 30 minutes. 30 days.

LOUISE: Every day I wait at least thirty minutes on the kids – at school – dropping them off ... picking them up. Thirty minutes here...thirty minutes there...it adds up.

MIA: That's amazing.

Excerpt from the play <u>Waiting for Oprah</u> by Mary Miller

January 25th

Act Now: Unexpected Acts of Love

Look for unexpected happiness in unexpected acts of kindness and unexpected acts of love. What do I mean? Think about it this way, we're so accustomed to looking for and finding what we expect that we are often disappointed, even when we get what we expect. Why? Because what we expect ... is just that ... it's what we expect. Instead look for the unexpected because it's in the unexpected that our lives are changed!

DORIE: Oh my God? What happened?

JOHN: Looks like we stopped.

DORIE: Why?

JOHN: We seem to be stuck.

Excerpt from the play <u>Ferris Wheel</u> by Mary Miller

January 26th

Setting the Stage

One of the reasons live theatre has survived through the centuries is the thrill of seeing people acting out a part right in front of you. The intimacy of theatre connects you with people. If you can see it acted on stage you realize you are not alone. You can identify with others. You can begin a conversation – a dialogue – and you begin to heal. But how do you change the stage you're on? You can begin by simply getting up and walking out of the room. Moving physically is the first step to moving mentally. They say (the experts) that it's hard to stay depressed when your body is in motion. So, get out of bed and off the couch and take a walk outside! You change your set, you change the scenery, you can change your life!

MAN: You need to see a shrink.

WOMAN: I have seen a shrink.

MAN: What did they say?

WOMAN: They said I should exert my authority.

Excerpt from the play Patterson's by Mary Miller

January 27th

Setting the Stage: Deja vu - you!

You are the designer in your own life. You can create any stage that you want. You can begin by stepping off the stage you're on and stepping onto the stage you want! This may sound confusing but it's not. It may sound hard but it's not. You can start by rearranging the furniture. At the Mary Miller Theatre we had one floor plan that we used for every play. No one ever noticed that it was the same design. They were always amazed at how different it looked! How a diner became a living room ... a living room became an amusement park ... an amusement park became an unfinished house ... and so on and so on! We changed the colors, rearranged the furniture, hung different pictures. The floor plan was always the same but the place (and the plays) were totally different! Even the characters (drastically different from play to play) were often played by the same cast of actors. Get it? Try it! Rearrange the furniture in your life and see if that doesn't make a difference in how you see yourself.

GEORGE: For your information this is power dressing, like they wear in New York City. It's part of the new image I'm cultivating for this cafe.

FRANK: Cafe?

GEORGE: That's right. As of today, I'm renaming this place, it's no longer "Dunford's Diner" it's now the official "Home of the Light Cafe".

Excerpt from the play <u>Light Burgers</u> by Mary Miller

January 28th

Setting the Stage: A New Day

Hello! Are you listening? Because this is going to do more to change your life than anything I've said before. Ready? You can create your own day. You can wake up each morning and create the day you are going to have. You can wake up and decide whether it's going to be a good day or a bad day. So why not wake up each morning and say I'm going to have a good day ... then set out to have one! Anything you can imagine ... your brain can create. Today really is the first day of the rest of your life!

JANICE: Oh Louise, you look great! I like your hair so much better with a perm!

LOUISE: (stunned) You do!?!

JANICE: It amazes me every time I see you.

LOUISE: (embarrassed) It amazes me every time I see it.

Excerpt from the play Waiting for Oprah by Mary Miller

January 29ᵗʰ

What play are you living?

The first thing we have to do to find out more about ourselves is to discover what type of play we are living: drama, comedy, or tragedy? Sometimes it's all three! Or is your life more like a mystery or detective story? Are you a long running saga like a soap opera or a thirty-minute sitcom? It's important to define the play you're living before you can change the story. If it's a tragedy try to figure out ways to interject a sense of humor. If it's a long running saga see if you can't foresee an ending that would benefit everyone. If it's a slapstick comedy interject a bit of pathos to add an element of poignancy and love. We all are living in our own play surrounded on stage by a cast of characters we call family. You may not be able to change the cast but you can always change the genre.

MERRILLEE: (panicked) You don't think those people out there have guns too, do you? I remember the movie The Day the Earth Stood Still the aliens landed in peace but the people shot 'em anyway. My teacher told me it was a metaphor, for our inability to accept anything different, but the aliens still left!

Excerpt from the play Light Burgers by Mary Miller

January 30th

On second thought!

It's not your first thought that counts ... it's your second thought! First thoughts can be misleading and wrong. Unfortunately they can make a lasting impression that's hard to overcome. You've heard the expression "you never get a second chance to make a good first impression" ... it may be true but it isn't right! A good play gives an actor a second chance to make a good first impression every night ... even after the play has been running for years! Life is like that if you're lucky to live long enough. You'll learn that your first thought is just that ... your first thought. It's your second thought that has real meaning. In life we rush too much and in the rushing we miss a lot. Sometimes the truth is found when we stop to take a second look.

JOHN: Are you sure you're all right?

DORIE: I'm fine. Couuuldn't be better.

JOHN: But you're not looking?

DORIE: No. Heights. I'm frightened of heights.

JOHN: And you ride a Ferris wheel?

Excerpt from the play <u>Ferris Wheel</u> by Mary Miller

January 31ˢᵗ

Second Thoughts on Aging

"If aging is all in the mind, how old are you? In your mind?" That's a line from my play, *A Christmas House* and it gets a laugh every time! When I talk about age, however, I don't mean your chronological age, I mean your mental age. Ask yourself does your mental age match your physical age? Keeping physically fit is important. That goes without saying. Getting your blood circulating helps both your body and your mind. The best actors are often in the best physical shape because acting can be grueling. But how do we age smarter? The answer is not so much about controlling your age (which you can't) as controlling your reaction to aging (which you can!). I have a good friend who practically went into cardiac arrest the day she turned 60! The day before she was fine. The day after she almost had a nervous breakdown. Nothing had changed physically except she was a day older. Mentally she suddenly became an old woman. This does not have to happen. The fact is no matter how old you are your brain continues to grow. We used to think everything with our brain stopped after the age of five ... that is not true! The brain cells you killed in college can grow back!! It just takes passion! A passion for living! And that passion will keep you young ... regardless of how old you happen to be!

BERNICE: I can't afford to spend extra money on something as foolish as acting!

CLARICE: You can't afford to just shrivel up and die! (pause) It was an old dream, wasn't it? But it's not dead yet. Is it?

Excerpt from the play Mulberry Lane by Mary Miller

February 1st

Second Thoughts on Worry

One of the poems I had to memorize as a child was "If" by Rudyard Kipling. "If you can keep your head when all about you are losing theirs...?" is the opening line and it's always struck me as a question of control. So often we seek to control those things around us, which we have no control over! It's a futile effort at best and yet we engage in it day after day. It consumes our time, our lives, and our world. It's time to stop worrying about things we cannot control like: world events, natural disasters, wars, and weather. How? By re-writing your script and asking yourself if your worrying about it will change it in any way? If the answer is no ... stop. Focus on what you can change and let the other go; then my friend, as the poems goes ... "Yours is the Earth and everything that's in it."

ANNE: Most of the time there's nothing wrong.

JOAN: But what if there is?

CLAIRE: (with a calming sense of authority) Then they'll fix it. If they find it here ... early like this. They'll fix it. So, don't worry. (Claire reaches out and takes Joan by the hand) You'll be fine. We'll all be fine.

Excerpt from the play <u>NEXT</u> by Mary Miller

February 2nd

Second Thoughts on Stress

Stress is killing us! Literally. A little bit every day. Learn to let it go. Stress is the key issue of our times. When you think about it stress will make you sick ... all that negative energy just churns through our body and makes us ill. We are what we think we are ... but what are we thinking? Look in the mirror. Do you love what you see? Do you even like what you see? Chances are you don't even recognize what you see! That's the toll stress takes on our body and our mind. It robs us of our vitality. I looked up the definition of stress in the dictionary: any event or circumstance in life that requires a person to adapt or change. Stress is change. It's as simple as that. The world is changing and we're stressed out! It's funny ... if you think about it. That's the one thing we can all agree on! So close your eyes, take a deep breath, realize you're not alone ... and smile. You'll be letting go of stress!

ALLISON: They say, "people who watch Oprah are more stressed out."

JANICE: Who told you that?

ALLISON: I read it.

LOUISE: That Oprah stresses people out?!

ALLISON: She dwells on stressful topics. Love. Peace. Spirituality. Weight!

FRAN: That stresses people out.

Excerpt from the play Waiting for Oprah by Mary Miller

February 3rd

Second Thoughts on Dialogue

What we say is important on stage and in life. Saying all those kind - wonderful - positive - life affirming things are great! But they don't change your life if you don't believe them. You can try and try but when you doubt yourself, mere words won't make a difference. That's why when you write the dialogue for your new life, write it in a way that you can actually believe it. If you are not thin, don't make your mantra "I am thin." Your mind won't believe it, and, every time you say it, your mind will counter with something like: "No you're not! You're fat." Which of course will only re-affirm the negativity you are trying to get rid of. Understand? So instead of starting your dialogue with "I am" begin with the words "I will." Feel the difference. I will is something you are going to do, be, and feel. The mind can grasp the concept of the future and will work with you to achieve it. It's not so much *acting* as *being.* You are going to be thin, be successful, be rich, be happy! Say "I will" and then set about making it happen.

MERRILLEE: *When the light comes ... will you look up at it? (pause) So I'll know I'm not crazy.*

L.E.: *You're not crazy.*

MERRILLEE: *But if it comes...*

L.E.: *(interrupting/goes to her) When it comes. You've got to stay positive now. I'm going to turn this radio on; you keep an ear out now. Maybe they'll announce something about where it's been spotted.*

Excerpt from the play Light Burgers by Mary Miller

February 4th

Second Thoughts on Sleep

As I am writing this I'm not getting any ... sleep. Sleep is the most underrated but necessary event in our lives and none of us get enough of it. It's the bane of our existence. Lack of sleep will literally drive you crazy. It's a form of torture that works. A lack of sleep can lead to illness and death! So how do you get to sleep ... when the minute you put your head down on the pillow your eyes open up? The thing I've found about sleep is the more I try to force myself to sleep ... the more awake I become. My brain wakes up at 3:00 o'clock in the morning and if I pause to acknowledge that fact, I never get back to sleep. Sound familiar? So if you can't get back to sleep by acting like you're asleep ... how do you avoid that 3:00 o'clock wake up call? You begin by realizing that it's normal. The idea that we get eight hours of sleep straight through the night is a myth. It's simply not true and striving for it only makes it harder to sleep. Instead of panicking when you wake up ... relax, roll over, and realize it's normal. Nine times out of ten, you'll be asleep before you know it; and chances are you'll forget you ever woke up. That's the beauty of most sleeping aids, they have an 'amnesia' effect that causes you to forget that you tossed and turned during the night! You're not sleeping better, you're just remembering less. So when you wake up ... don't freak out ... it's just part of the normal sleep pattern. Close your eyes and turn off your brain. Sweet dreams...

PEARL: When I was your age, I used to sleep like a baby. Now days seems I be lucky to get two or three hours all toll? And when I do fall off I keep having this dream. I'm in this house but I'm packing to leave. I don't know where I'm going but I'm packing just the same.

Excerpt from the play I Witness by Mary Miller

35

February 5ᵗʰ

Stress and Multitasking ... or ... You can't play two parts on the same stage at the same time.

Multitasking is impossible! Let me say that again ... multitasking is impossible. It is physically impossible to do two things at the same time. Don't kid yourself. If you are multitasking then you are doing multiple tasks badly. And you'll probably end up having to do one or more tasks all over again to get them right! Picture a stage ... now imagine trying to play two parts at the same time ... you can't do it! Your audience will walk out!! The same is true in life. Take a moment to focus on one task at a time, finish that task and then focus on the next, again and again. Your stress level will decrease, your productivity will increase, and you will never run the risk of losing the audience.

BERNICE: Hello, my name is Bernice Pendergrast and for my audition I will be portraying Juliet, from Shakespeare's Romeo and Juliet... O Romeo, Romeo, wherefore art thou Romeo? Deny thy father and refuse thy name, or, if thou wilt not, be but sworn my love, and I'll no longer be a Capulet.

CLARICE: (clapping) You're going to be wonderful.

Excerpt from the play Mulberry Lane by Mary Miller

February 6th

Dare to be happy!

I double dog dare you!! Sometimes I think people are so afraid to be happy that they embrace pain. Pain can feel comfortable because, if you've lived long enough, you've experienced pain. And it hurts ... but you can get use to it. You can get used to almost anything if you put your mind to it. But why get used to pain? Why not reach out for happiness? People say pain is real and happiness is an illusion. Who made these rules? It is so much easier as a writer to make an audience cry than it is to make them laugh. It's a fact. Ask any actor ... comedy is hard!! So get to work. Smile. Be happy! Misery has enough company ... dare to be happy!

ALLISON: I just wanted everything to look nice for our last meeting.

LOUISE: Don't say that! It just makes me sad. I don't want to be sad. Not today. Not with Oprah coming and all...

(The doorbell rings and they both jump.)

Excerpt from the play <u>Waiting for Oprah</u> by Mary Miller

February 7ᵗʰ

Setting the stage: What, me change?

People talk a lot about change. Especially changing someone else! But the question I hear is: "Do I need to change? What is wrong with staying the same?" Nothing really, except it's harder than you think. Even if you are not changing ... the world is changing. Events around you are changing at a faster clip than ever before. Does that matter? Does that affect your life? I don't know. Do you dread getting up in the morning? Do you dread going to work? Do you dread coming home? These are obvious signs that you need a change. But a more subtle and telling question to ask is: Are you bored? A sign of boredom is a sign to change.

MATTIE: Some people are opposed to change no matter how much more convenient it'd be.

CHANDLER: Some people are just scared of change.

ADELE: Some people don't embrace it as readily as others.

Excerpt from the play <u>Virgin Tears</u> by Mary Miller

February 8ᵗʰ

Setting the stage: What, me worry?

When you spend your life worrying you can miss life all together! The problem with worry is that 90% of the time we worry about things that never ... I repeat .... never happen. In that sense we waste real time, energy, and joy! No matter how much you worry about the past, you can't change it. No matter how much you worry about the future, you don't know what it will be. No matter how much you worry about the moment, this too will pass. The KEY is to determine if what you are worried about is really worth worrying about. If it is ... take action. If it is not ... you guessed it ... stop worrying. Clear the stage and your mind of worry and get on with the show and your life!!

LIZBETH: Momma, I'm a grown woman. You don't have to worry about me.

ABIGAIL: A grown woman my foot. You are my baby and you'll always be my baby, and as long as you are under my roof ... (she looks up) ... which is the only thing this house seems to have, I'm going to worry!

Excerpt from the play <u>A Christmas House</u> by Mary Miller

February 9th

Walking across the stage! ... or ... How do I get from here to there?

Sometimes the hardest thing to do is to start. The law of inertia states that a body at rest tends to stay at rest. So how do you get from here to there? The best way to begin is to start by saying "yes." Say yes to things that move you in the direction you want to go. We can often visualize where we would like to end up ... but seeing a path to get there can be hard. Most of the time there's no clear-cut path ... no yellow brick road! I think one of the things that's so appealing about the *Wizard of Oz* is the simplicity of following the yellow brick road! So, if you start by saying "yes" and put one foot in front of the next, you never know where you might end up. In an interview Ringo Star was asked how he became one of the Beatles. His answer was he said "yes" to everything they asked him. He wanted to be in a band, they asked him, he said yes, and the rest is history!

L.E.: (trying to understand) Merrillee even if that light was a UFO, and it had been calling you, and was going to take you with it; why would you consider going off with some stranger to some place you don't even know?

MERRILLEE: Because I was invited.

Excerpt from the play <u>Light Burgers</u> by Mary Miller

February 10th

Make new friends.

There is an old song I learned as a Girl Scout: "Make new friends but keep the old ones ... one is silver and the other is gold." I always thought it was a little sappy ... overly sentimental ... and childish. Until I got old enough to appreciate it. Old enough to have both old friends and new friends. Now, I'm not sure the song is sentimental enough! When we're young we take making friends for granted. It's easy. We're all experiencing the same thing, have a lot in common, and willing to go an extra mile for one another. But as we get older we grow more insular ... more protective ... more solitary. We have families of our own and they take up a good deal of our time, whether we like them or not! We don't have time to make new friends. But it's important in this game of life to bring new players on to your stage. It takes more work to make friends when you are older. But it's worth it and in my opinion it's even more important. You can never replace the old friends in your life but you can make new ones ... and they are both golden.

MIA: We're more than a book club.

LOUISE: We're like a family.

JANICE: A dysfunctional family.

ALLISON: I wouldn't call us dysfunctional. We have issues.

JANICE: People without issues are medicated!

Excerpt from the play <u>Waiting for Oprah</u> by Mary Miller

February 11th

Acting Happy: Create a Memory

One of the best ways to be happy is to create a happy memory. How? Do something fun! Right now!! You don't have to go on a vacation ... you don't have to wait for a special occasion. It doesn't have to be an expensive adventure. You don't even have to leave the house. But you do have to plan to do something out of the ordinary. Something special. Something fun. By taking time out of your day to create a happy memory you give yourself a gift you can reopen anytime especially on those dark rainy days when everything is gloomy and happiness seems beyond your reach. You can take a trip back to that happy memory and re-live it all over again. It's free. It's fun. It lasts a lifetime. Happiness isn't something you find ... it's something you make.

CHANDLER: That's it! That's what we need to do reconstruct the Merry MAC and sail out of this old town.

MATTIE: In a cardboard box with a pink bed sheet sail?

CHANDLER: Why not? I used to think that boat could take us anywhere.

MATTIE: Don't you think we are a little too old to set sail in the Merry MAC?

CHANDLER: You're never too old to set sail in an imaginary boat!

Excerpt from the play <u>Virgin Tears</u> by Mary Miller

February 12th

How do you do ... the things you do?

How do you make Acting Healthy work for your life's play? How do you step off the stage you are on ... and step onto the stage you want ... without falling into the orchestra pit?! Let your passion be your guide. Years ago Joseph Campbell said to follow your bliss. He was right. But I'll take it a step further; to truly succeed in changing your life's script you have to have more motivation than 'bliss' ... you have to have passion. I don't care what your passion is, passion is the driving force in all change. Passion is the 'how' in this theatrical adventure I call life. Passion is what wakes you up in the morning, brings you back to life, and gives you a reason to live. Passion is the answer.

CLARICE: *(proudly) I had my moments on stage.*

BERNICE: *You can't live off moments.*

CLARICE: *You can't live without 'em!*

Excerpt from the play <u>Mulberry Lane</u> by Mary Miller

February 13th

Grabbing victory out of the jaws of defeat.

Sometimes no matter what you do things goes wrong. You walk across the stage and the scenery falls over for no reason and you are standing there exposed to the elements not having a clue as to what to do or how to rectify the situation. There is no way you can pretend that it didn't happen. There is no amount of acting that is going to keep the audience from noticing. The best thing for you to do in a case like this ... is just sit back and laugh. Your audience will love you for it! They will laugh with you. They will remember you forever. The same is true in life. When everything around you seems to be going wrong, you have a choice, you can either laugh or cry. Why not laugh! The best way to grab victory out of the jaws of defeat is to laugh ... because if you can still laugh, you are not defeated!

LOUISE: When Oprah gets here ... I'd like to ask her why?

FRAN: Why there's pain?

MIA: Why there's suffering?

ALLISON: Why good things happen to bad people?

JANICE: Why you can't wear white after Labor Day?

Excerpt from the play Waiting for Oprah by Mary Miller

February 14th

Happy Valentine's Day

On Valentine's Day most of the focus is on couples, which is great if you are a couple but it can be downright depressing if you are not. The thing that I've found, however, that is more important than being able to say "I love you" to someone else ... is to say "I love you" to yourself. This Valentine's Day stand in front of a mirror and look at your reflection and say "I love you" and say it until you mean it! After all you are the great love of your life. Learn to love yourself and you will be better able to love someone else ... any day of the year.

JOHN: (covering) Yeah, well, you get used to being alone. You get over it. You adjust.

DORIE: Isn't that the truth. Why, I don't even mind eating by myself anymore. Not as long as I have something to read. Newspaper, magazine, those little bitty sugar packets they set at the table, the ones with the history of each state written real tiny on the back. You can learn a lot eating alone. The state flowers. The state birds ...

(Suddenly he leans over and kisses her on the cheek.)

Excerpt from the play <u>Ferris Wheel</u> by Mary Miller

February 15th

Discovering your character.

The beauty of acting is the fact that you don't have to be yourself. If you want to bring more joy in your life, act like a happy person. If you want more empathy, act with compassion. If you want to be thinner, act thin! You don't have to worry about winning the academy award ... your goal is to discover the character you want to be and learn to play the part.

CLARICE: Here it is! Open auditions for their upcoming season. (reading) As You Like It. Romeo & Juliet. Arsenic and Old Lace. Member of the Wedding...

BERNICE: Arsenic and Old Lace?

CLARICE: You'd be perfect! There are at least two or three parts for women over sixty!

BERNICE: I remember that show. It came through town after you left and I went to see it with Daddy. We acted out the parts for weeks. Momma thought we were crazy but I loved that show.

Excerpt from the play <u>Mulberry Lane</u> by Mary Miller

February 16th

Picture the part.

Picture yourself as a character in your life's play (it's easier to make changes that way.) Keep in mind, however, that some parts of your life cannot be recast and some parts of your stage cannot be rebuilt. What you can change is the dialogue, supporting cast, costumes, hair, makeup, etc.! Beginning to get the picture? I'm not talking about radically changing everything in your life. I'm talking about systematically changing some things. Look at your life as a play and it's easy to see where you've made mistakes. Now an even better exercise is to look at you life as a *future* play and picture where you want to end up. The future is yet to be written. Picture the part you want to play, cast yourself in it, and start living that life today.

MERRILLEE: (CONT.) I wonder what ever happened to that big pink shell. You don't have it do you Lenora Elaine?

L.E.: Now what would I do with a big pink conch shell?!

MERRILLEE: You never know what people save. Why I found a whole pile of old Lady's Home Journals down in Mamma's basement you know the magazines with those questionnaire articles like "How Much Do You Love?" "Can This Marriage Be Saved?" "Rate Yourself as a Lover". I tell you if you answer those questions truly they can give you a whole lot of insight into your personality you never knew you had.

Excerpt from the play Light Burgers by Mary Miller

February 17th

Bigger than life.

The characters we love on stage and in film tend to be bigger than life. They play their parts with enthusiasm that demands you watch them. You can't take your eyes off of them, even when they are not saying a word. These are people who understand that life is a gift and they live it to the fullest. My grandmother was like that ... bigger than life ... and she inspired in me the joy of living. To this day, I don't know anyone who didn't love "Big Anne." Even her name was Big! Big Anne never dwelt on the negative and *nothing* was impossible. She was a role model for me before I even understood what a role model was. Big Anne was bigger than life. She played her part with enthusiasm and love. Bring that same enthusiasm to your life. Play your part boldly. Dare to live bigger.

UPSTAIRS: There are no guarantees to anything. It's a brave new world.

DOWNSTAIRS: No, it's not. It's the same old shitty place it's always been. Only now it's getting worse and this won't prove anything.

UPSTAIRS: It will too! It'll prove I was here. That I existed. My name will be written down and people will see it. The Guinness Book of World Records is published in every language imaginable, all recording the ultimate achievements of man.

Excerpt from the play <u>At 3:00 O'clock in the Morning</u> by Mary Miller

February 18th

Get to the point!

Every good story has a beginning, middle, and *end.* So when you are talking to other people remember to get to the end of your story quickly! Brevity is the sole of wit! Sometimes we get so caught up in our own story we forget that other people have stories to tell too! The best way to make friends and influence people is to listen. On stage it's called 'active listening' ... the ability to actively listen to information as if you were hearing it for the very first time. Active listening is the same in life. Listen to what others have to say and respond accordingly. A play where one character dominates the stage is boring. Be the person who brightens a room when they enter it ... not when they leave it! Get to the point of your story and actively listen to what other people have to say ... and you will always be the life of the party!!

JOHN: I'd have thought anybody as ... ah ... as ... chatty ... as you would have won Miss Congeniality.

DORIE: That's just my breeding. My Mother always said it was our social obligation to be entertaining.

JOHN: Don't have to feel any obligation on my account!!

Excerpt from the play <u>Ferris Wheel</u> by Mary Miller

February 19th

Thinking from the heart.

Instead of thinking from the head ... try thinking from the heart. Focus on compassion, empathy, and love. True greatness really comes from an outpouring of the heart. So, why are we so fixated on the head? Why do we believe that things from the heart are naive? Sometimes, I guess it's just easier. To act from the heart means you really have to consider the consequences of your actions ... you really have to engage with one another. We don't engage much anymore. Not really. We stay in touch with Facebook and Twitter and e-mails and blogs etc ... but we rarely engage one another from the heart. If we did it might be a better world ... it would certainly be a better place to live. Maybe that's the place to start ... thinking from the heart.

CHILD: But I love you.

WOMAN: That ain't enough. Child ... child, you gots to love me so much that the only color you see is the color of my heart. And I got to love you the same. And we got to take proper care to treat people right, that's the only way we be able to live together ... you and me and Mary Lou O'Callahan ...

Excerpt from the play Take Proper Care by Mary Miller

February 20th

Stage managing sleep.

Have you ever been so tired you couldn't sleep? Why is it that when we lay our head down on our pillow and finally allow ourselves to sleep ... sleep is the last thing that comes? I think it's a multitude of things. A multitude of people, places, and events that come at us at an ever increasing rate. It's like being on stage and every few minutes someone changes the script. I used to work on the soap opera "All My Children" and it wasn't unusual for the director or writer or producer to come down to the set and hand you a new script. Suddenly your character would make 360 degree turn ... and you had to learn the lines and act the part all in a matter of minutes. That's how fast life can change. And I think it is keeping us up at night. Sometimes we don't know when it's 'safe' to go to sleep, because something is always happening somewhere. Maybe we're afraid that some unseen director or writer or producer is preparing new pages for us. It is enough to keep you up at night unless you realize that life really is more like a sound stage than not. In the morning the lights go up and the show goes on. But at night after the audience has left and the stage is empty ... I picture a stage manager quietly turning off the lights, telling everyone to go home, and get a good nights rest. Something about that thought is enough to give me permission to turn off my brain and go to sleep.

CLARICE: Bernice, there are people here who would have been dead years ago if it wasn't for your snoring. I should get a tape recording and send it off to Ripley's Believe It Or Not. Or better yet the American Medical Society. Miss Bernice Pendergrast asleep in F flat. Snnnnnooooorrrr.

Excerpt from the play <u>Mulberry Lane</u> by Mary Miller

February 21st

Half full?

The first thing that comes to mind when people talk about positive thinking is the age-old question: Is your glass half full or half empty? There are dissertations done over the response to this question. People have pondered it for years. Scientists and psychologists can produce charts and grafts to show you exactly where you fit in the spectrum of well-being depending on your answer. And those knowing friends who officiously ask you, when you are having a particularly bad day, if your glass is half full or half empty, run the risk of having you throw whatever is in your glass in their face! And therein lies the real answer to the question. Because it's not whether you have a glass that is half full or half empty that makes a difference in your life; it's the fact that you have a glass at all to begin with that makes the difference in everyone's life. How you choose to fill that glass is up to you. But if you begin with the realization that you have a glass you are light years ahead of the person trying to figure out if it's half empty or half full.

ROBERT: Chandler, wait! (She stops and looks back at him. He is suddenly hesitant ... nervous ... as he weighs his words.) Now that you mention it, there is ... something ... I'd like to ask you?

CHANDLER: What?

ROBERT: First have another glass of champagne. (Robert takes the champagne and pours her another glass.)

Excerpt from the play <u>Virgin Tears</u> by Mary Miller

February 22nd

Reaching for the stars.

When reaching for the stars ... how do you do it? Do you stand on a chair? Go to the top floor of the tallest building? Climb a mountain? I know reaching for the stars is a metaphorical phrase. But I'm talking about literally reaching up for something that is beyond your grasp. And it may sound strange where I believe we get our best leg up. It's not by ourselves, of course. It's not by good intentions, although those can help. It's not even so much by someone reaching back to pull you up, as good as that can be. But how high we go and how much we achieve, I think, is in direct proportion to the size of the obstacle in front of us. The old expression: What doesn't kill me makes me stronger. Is never truer than it is here. Without that obstacle in front of you, you might never know how high you can reach. In a strange but true way ... what's in your way may give you the best leg up in achieving your goals. A launching pad to shoot for the stars.

JOHN: Your knuckles are turning white. Are you sure this is good for your circulation?

DORIE: What doesn't kill me makes me stronger, type of thing.

JOHN: So you do this in lieu of a birthday party with cake and ice cream?

DORIE: Oh no, I have that too, when I get through. Like a reward.

Excerpt from the play Ferris Wheel by Mary Miller

February 23rd

Darkest before the dawn.

That's what they say: it's darkest before the dawn. I don't know why it's true. I suppose it's because we hope it's true. Sometimes when it's darkest we can't help but hope that it will get lighter. And if you wait long enough it generally does. Slowly but surely. That's the thing I like best about live theatre ... it can condense a lifetime into an evening's performance. You can watch actors on stage plumb to depths that you'd never like to go in real life. But from the safe distance of the audience you can watch in the dark and learn how they navigate those deep waters. Sometimes it can be a perfect blueprint for your life. Other times it just serves as a reminder that things change ... and change isn't always bad. Sometimes change is just change and darkness is just darkness ... and if you leave in the middle of the show, you'll never know how the play ends. Hang in there ... it's always darkest before the dawn.

ALLISON: I wish you had told us.

FRAN: I haven't told anyone. Talking about it just makes it worse. There's nothing you can do.

LOUISE: I bet Oprah can do something.

FRAN: I wish she could.

Excerpt from the play <u>Waiting for Oprah</u> by Mary Miller

February 24th

Take a chance.

To make a change you have to take a chance. Buy a ticket. Get on board. Make a move. One thing I know for sure, to borrow a phrase from Oprah, is that the only way to change your life is to take a chance on life. And that means taking a chance on you. Most of the time we are afraid to change because we are afraid of failing. But not trying is the only failure. If you have a dream it's never too late to act on it, in some form or fashion. You don't have to hit the Broadway stage to be an actor ... there are hundreds of community theatres begging for people to join them. You don't have to write the great American Novel to be a writer .... you can keep a journal, write a story, or post a letter. You don't have to be the best in the business to be the best you can be. And being your best, whether you succeed or fail, you win! Take a chance ... it's a sure bet.

MASON: Come on L.E. take a look. Take a chance.

L.E.: No.

MASON: Just one look?

L.E.: No.

(Mason holds his hand out to L.E., she doesn't move.)

MASON: What are you afraid of? Trust me.

Excerpt from the play Light Burgers by Mary Miller

February 25th

Things happen.

As much as we want to try and control our lives ... we can't. Not really. Not in the long run. In the long run ... things happen. Good and bad. Of course, we rarely talk about the good. Good things are what we expect ... what we deserve. But bad things do happen and they happen to good people. Whether it's bad news, bad health, bad weather ... things happen. And I refuse to simplify it all by saying *bad things help us appreciate good things* because it's not true in the moment. It may be true later, but in that moment when you get bad news what helps is to take a moment, take a breath, take stock of what is good, and use that as a starting point to deal with ... bad news, bad health, and bad weather. Because things happen.

UPSTAIRS: You've been a teller for twenty-five years?

DOWNSTAIRS: An Account Management Supervisor!

UPSTAIRS: I've never known anyone to work anywhere for twenty-five years in a row.

DOWNSTAIRS: It happens. I received my certificate for loyal service in the mail today.

UPSTAIRS: Congratulations!

DOWNSTAIRS: It came with a pink slip.

Excerpt from the play <u>At 3:00 O'clock in the Morning</u> by Mary Miller

February 26th

Tired so tired.

Sometimes you just have to take a break ... stop what you are doing ... and put your head down. Remember in Kindergarten we'd bring a little rug to class and everybody would take a nap. Then in Middle School we'd put our heads down on the desk while the teacher read to us from the front of the room. When we were little it seems like we were encouraged to take naps; now you'll be fired for sleeping on the job. Funny thing is, as a kid, I don't remember needing a nap! But I sure do now!! I'd love to take a little rug and lie down for a moment at work. In Spain they call it a *siesta*. It's a tradition we'd do well to adopt. It seems no one here is getting enough sleep these days and it's making us all angry. Angry at the world. Angry at work. Angry at ourselves. Anger on stage can be a good thing but in life can be devastating. Nowadays it feels as if we're constantly at war but we're not sure who the enemy is, so we fight with everyone and that anger is eating us up alive and keeping us up at night. Maybe it's time to take a break ... stop what you are doing ... and put your head down and rest.

DOWNSTAIRS: It's 3:00 o'clock in the morning! You can't keep walking around your apartment at 3:00 o'clock in the morning!!

UPSTAIRS: It's my apartment.

DOWNSTAIRS: But I hear every move you make! This afternoon I tried to ignore it. At 10:00 o'clock I thought I could sleep through it. By midnight I figured it would stop. But it hasn't and I can't.

Excerpt from the play At 3:00 O'clock in the Morning by Mary Miller

February 27ᵗʰ

Keep it to yourself.

We are sooooo eager to tell the world what we are doing that most of the time we never get around to doing it. Somehow when the word gets out, the excitement inside dies. I know a lot of writers, including myself, who won't tell you the end of a story until they've finished writing it. Even if I know full well how it ends. Because part of the thrill of writing is keeping that secret inside, and that secret can become a powerful motivating force, powerful enough to motivate you through to the end. So, if you want to reach a goal, any goal, don't tell people what you're doing ... just get out there and do it. Quietly. Without fanfare or expectation. You'll succeed more often than not! Why? Because by keeping it to yourself you don't have to worry about what other people think, say, or do. Best of all you don't have to worry about failing because no one knows you are trying ... except for you! And you can keep a secret, right?

MATTIE: Adele will be so happy to see you.

CHANDLER: You didn't tell her?

MATTIE: It's been almost two years, Chandler. I wasn't even sure you'd come back. I didn't want to disappoint her. She's been so disappointed before.

Excerpt from the play <u>Virgin Tears</u> by Mary Miller

February 28th

Splendor in the grass.

I was reading about a park in New York City that was not actually a park but an art gallery. Inside, instead of art on the walls, the gallery was filled with life-size replicas of trees and flowers and bushes and grass all in full bloom under a brilliant blue sky with scattered white clouds painted on the ceiling. A perfect reproduction of a beautiful park at the height of spring ... in the middle of winter. A place where winter weary New Yorkers could go and escape the harsh realities of the weather and experience a warm spring day during their lunch hour. A place where they could take picnic lunches and sit on artificial grass and roll up their sleeves to bathe in the sunlight that came from an overhead lightening system. The perfect theatrical stage! Nothing about it was real ... but something about it made a difference. People would go in depressed and come out happy. Even though they knew it wasn't spring, for a brief moment they felt like it was, and in that moment it made a difference in how they felt about the day. Spring is a state of mind. Keep your mind open. There is true splendor in the grass ... whether that grass is real or artificial.

GEORGE: Look at "Rock City" Tennessee. Have you ever seen "Rock City"? There ain't nothing to see there but rocks! What we have here is a real natural phenomenon and Mason says it's worth paying a dollar or two more for everything I got....

L.E.: Mason says! Mason says! Who cares what Mason says?!

GEORGE: He's been living in New York City!! Working in advertising. He knows the answers. And he's giving them to me for free.

Excerpt from the play <u>Light Burgers</u> by Mary Miller

February 29th (once every four years!)

Leap Year

In 1582 Pope Gregory XIII instituted the Gregorian calendar and established its first leap year in 1584. Why? Because a year is really longer than 365 days it's 365.2 days and to keep the seasons from bumping into each other Pope Gregory decided to add an extra day every four years. Amazing! Today is our extra day. Today we get 24 more hours than we did last year. For those born on February 29th it's time to celebrate. For the rest of us why not celebrate it too. When you think of all the things modern man has created few things can surpass creating another day!

JOHN: Happy birthday.

DORIE: Thank you.

Excerpt from the play Ferris Wheel by Mary Miller

March 1ˢᵗ

Sing your song.

In listening to k.d. lang sing Leonard Cohen's *Hallelujah* it brought tears to my eyes. All my life I have wished I could sing. I even took singing lessons in New York (a pure waste of time and money!) except for the fact that when I left I felt exhilarated. I'd walk down the streets of Manhattan to the subway with a song on my lips, which was OK in New York City because no one was listening to me! We like to think that people are watching us but most of the time they're not ... and they're really not in New York City! Everybody in that town seems to be marching to their own song. I was one of many. It was funny to me I had friends who had excellent voices but they rarely sang because they could tell the difference between a well-hit note and a sour one. I thought they were just too hard on themselves. Not me. I sang in the subway and on the train and all the way back home. I knew the notes were off but I sang anyway. Now I no longer live in New York and I no longer walk everywhere I go. More often than not I'm in a car. But I still love to roll the windows down and sing aloud ... a song for myself. Sing your song ... it doesn't have to be perfect to be good.

Back at the house the sun was setting. The girls had placed individual work lamps strategically to emit the most light through the 2x4 walls. As they worked, the three sisters san "We Three Kings" ... making up the words as they decorated the house for Christmas.

Excerpt from the book <u>A Christmas House</u> by Mary Miller

March 2nd

Gift of laughter.

As a writer the hardest thing to do is make someone laugh ... because laughter comes from deep down inside and catches you by surprise. In fact, I think that is the definition of comedy ... surprise. And it is a gift. The experts say people who laugh live longer, years longer than their counterparts. Laughing is actually considered good exercise. It burns calories and tightens the abdominal muscles. There is nothing about laughter that isn't good! It makes you happy. It makes those people around you happy. It's contagious. Have you ever started laughing because someone else was laughing? You don't even have to know why ... you just laugh. Laughter frees the soul in ways that tears do not. Laughter opens the heart when anger closes it. Laughter is the gateway to love. Laugh when you have the chance. Laugh out loud. Exercise those muscles. The more you laugh ... the more you're filled with joy. Make someone laugh today ... give them the gift of laughter and yourself the gift of joy.

ABIGAIL: What's so funny?

FRED: I was just thinking about our honeymoon. Remember in the middle of the night, you scream and I jumped like I'd been shot. I didn't know what happened.

ABIGAIL: I sat in the toilet bowl! You left the seat up! I grew up with girls. It was just Celeste and me. I didn't know what to expect.

FRED: You looked real pretty that night. (he smiles at her) Still do now.

Excerpt from the play <u>A Christmas House</u> by Mary Miller

March 3rd

Make a lasting impression.

Clichés are clichés because they have been proven over time. But clichés can be contradictory because life is more complicated than most clichés. "You never get a second chance to make a good first impression"...but ... "First impressions can be misleading." And people have many many many many faces. So, how do you make a lasting impression? The best way I've found is to make a positive impression first. What do I mean? When you meet someone for the first time, instead of solely focusing on their name (which is a good thing) but it is usually accomplished by linking their name with something bizarre that has nothing to do with them but triggers a connection in your brain that causes you to remember who they are. Instead when you see someone for the first time ... and I mean in that first 30 seconds ... think of something positive to say about them and say it! Compliment them and they will remember you!! Odds are you'll remember them too for exactly who they are because in that first 30 seconds you will have invested something of yourself ... and in that moment you'll make an impression that lasts.

MERRILLEE: Mamma used to say: "If you want to be welcomed, never go anywhere empty handed."

FRANK: Your Mamma sure was full of a lot of little expressions.

MERRILLEE: Social Rules of Life she called 'em. Said if you followed them, no matter what, your social life will always flourish.

Excerpt from the play <u>Light Burgers</u> by Mary Miller

March 4th

Writing as therapy.

You want to learn something about yourself? Keep a journal. It's easy ... once you get started. I don't know about you, but when I first open a blank journal I find it intimidating! That clean beautiful white sheet of paper staring up at me. I pause and wait for inspiration. I can't write something dumb on the first page of the book, people always read the first page of a book. (It may be the only page they read!) So I rack my brain trying to think of some brilliant thing to write. How about a quote?...but then a quote from whom?...and saying what? Should I write my name...should it be cursive or print? I sit there sweating, wondering where to start. Do I write in pencil or pen? What if I misspell a word? I don't want to look dumb! I'm sweating even more. Oh my gosh, what if they find it after I'm dead. Will they be able to read my writing? Will they want to publish it? Will I have accurately chronicled my times? Am I qualified to chronicle my times?! The pressure is immense!! Most people at this point close the journal, put it back on the shelf and say good riddance to the whole process!! And they leave frustrated and unenlightened. But I have the solution to that daunting first blank page. It's a simple solution. Simply turn the page and start on page two ... and leave the first page blank!

CHILD: There're good things too.

WOMAN: Well then, I'm counting on you to keep a record.

CHILD: I could do that. I could write 'em all down in a diary and tell you about 'em when I see you again.

Excerpt from the play <u>Take Proper Care</u> by Mary Miller

March 5th

Leading with strength.

Lead with your strengths. It should go without saying but theses days we spend so much time improving our weaknesses we forget about our strengths and that's wrong. Because when we actually lead with our strengths we thrive. People blossom when they are allowed and encouraged to do what they do best. They are enthusiastic, energetic, and passionate. You can spend hours improving your weaknesses and get pretty good ... but spend hours improving your strengths and you become great! Focus on what you like to do and build a career and a life around that. Let that be your life's play ... and let that play begin now.

ABIGAIL: What business?

MARGARET: Selling white chocolate candy at flea markets.

BABS: Margaret, will you stop it! Now Momma, let me explain, you know how I've always gotten so many compliments on the little things I make. Well, I decided wouldn't it be fun to set up a little business of my own making and selling all kinds of things?

Excerpt from the play <u>A Christmas House</u> by Mary Miller

March 6th

Laugh at yourself.

One of the most disarming things that you can do on stage to win your audience is to laugh ... especially if you are messing up! Just laugh. You might as well laugh first ... because if you laugh first, then everyone else will be laughing with you and not at you. Sometimes we take ourselves so seriously that we stop ourselves from laughing. This is probably the worst thing we could do and it's usually at the worst possible time. Laughter releases stress. Laughter enables us to move on from point A to point B. If you can laugh at yourself you give yourself permission not only to fail but permission to try again. Remember life is meant to be enjoyed ... give yourself permission to laugh ... and laugh at yourself! Because if you can laugh at yourself you'll win over the world.

(Suddenly a fourth woman, Anne, bursts into the room. She is hurried and tying her identical seersucker gown around her waist as she enters. She looks at Claire then at Barbara.)

ANNE: Hi. (to Claire) Hey. (to Barbara) You here for a mammogram? (she smiles, no one answers but they nod.)   I should have figured...unless of course it's a spend-the-night party!? (she pulls at her seersucker top) One size fits all. Now that is a joke. (she laughs at herself) I got lost. (pause) From the bathroom. All the rooms look alike. (she laughs again) Don't want to be sitting in the wrong room. No telling what test they'll run on you!

Excerpt from the play <u>NEXT</u> by Mary Miller

March 7ᵗʰ

SPIT IT OUT!!

You can do that you know! You can throw food away. Whoever said we had to clean our plates to feed the starving children in China was mistaken. Your cleaning your plate will have no effect on anyone in China (or anywhere else for that matter!) If you insist on eating a whole delicious cake...share it with the universe: eat a piece, throw away a piece, eat a piece. Get the picture? Oh, you can't do that, you say. Why not? You don't want to waste it. But isn't that what you're doing when you eat the whole thing? Aren't you wasting it? We were way past "hungry" with the meal we had before we even sat down to dessert! You can throw it away that cookie you have in your hand, look at it, figure out why you are eating it ... if you are not really hungry, throw it away. Confuse your brain. It cannot understand the concept of famine (diet!) if you are throwing away the super deluxe homemade chocolate chip cookie. Trust me. And if you can't throw it away, save it for another day or another person. Most of us are not hungry. Eat to feel full, not to feel love.

BABS: So? The other day he walks into the house eats a piece of the roof of the nativity crèche and then he wonders why I'm so upset. Do you have any idea how long I slave over a hot stove melting all that white chocolate down, adding just the right amount of food coloring 'til it gets the perfect shade, pour it into those molds, wait for it to dry, then carefully, ever so carefully peel it out so it won't break--just to have him come in, pop it into his mouth and ask "What's for dinner, honey?" I swear I thought I'd die. I grabbed him by the throat and shouted "Spit it out! Spit it out!!" I had to reach down into his mouth and pull it out before he ruined everything.

Excerpt from the play <u>A Christmas House</u> by Mary Miller

March 8ᵗʰ

It takes time.

In this world where everything is instant ... including instant gratification ... it's important to take a moment to realize that good things take time. Not everything can be rushed. Sometimes it takes years to materialize ... years to mature. We know *good wine takes time* Ernest & Julio Gallo told us that! But sometimes it just takes time to appreciate and even recognize the truly good things we have surrounding us. If you are healthy that is a good thing. If you have a place to live that is a good thing. If you have a job that is a good thing too. But all these things take time. And sometimes we just have to wait, which isn't easy in this hurry up world. Yes, it takes time, but most of the time ... the wait is worth it.

FRED: Abby, building a house takes time.

ABIGAIL: It takes time? IT TAKES TIME!! If I hear "it takes time" one more time I'm going to scream. Fred, do you realize, it's Christmas Eve and our entire family is coming here to spend Christmas with us! What are we going to do? You deliberately led me to believe this house was finished!

FRED: It's almost finished.

Excerpt from the play <u>A Christmas House</u> by Mary Miller

March 9th

War & Peace

The biggest conflict on stage is the conflict between war and peace, whether that is portrayed as a family dinner or an international incident. On stage it is important to have an enemy you can fight against and win to have a satisfying night of theatre. But in life that battle is never so easily won, nor is it always so clear as to who is the good guy and who is the bad guy. Such is the drama of life. As much as conflict is the driving engine on stage conflict in life can tear a person apart. I'm not advocating avoiding conflict in life, I'm just advocating seeking a more peaceful solution to solve your life's problems. Once in the thick of battle, we often wonder why we started fighting in the first place. War is chaotic and messy. Battles on stage are exciting but they are also carefully thought out and choreographed. If they are well played they appear to be real and it's thrilling. Peace on stage is boring. But peace in life is invigorating. As much as theatre can mirror life, in this case, it's mirror opposites. In life seek peace. On stage give yourself permission to embrace all the conflict you can stand because at the end of the night, the curtain will come down and life (hopefully a peaceful one) will resume.

ADELE: I hated you for leaving! I wondered how you escaped?

CHANDLER: I didn't escape, Adele. I just ran the other way.

(They stand at opposite ends of the stage, looking at each other for the first time. There is a moment of recognition between them.)

ADELE: You can stop now, if you want to. You can stop running.

Excerpt from the play <u>Virgin Tears</u> by Mary Miller

March 10th

A job well done.

"JOB WELL DONE." These are three of the most coveted words in the English language, next to "I love you." I don't care who you are or where you are from when you strive to do a good job and succeed, you want some recognition. You need a pat on the back. It's not enough to simply say it yourself ... someone else has to recognize it too and applaud you for your efforts. This is where a good teacher or a good friend comes into play. Someone who knows you and respects you. Someone who will mean it when they say it ... and you will believe it when you hear it! It's the applause at the end of a show. It's taking that extra bow. We all need recognition sometime in our life in order to move forward. Find someone who has done a good job and congratulate them ... tell them today it was a job well done!

BERNICE: I'll have you know I got a great deal of satisfaction out of doing my job well. Those people appreciated me. They needed me...

Excerpt from the play <u>Mulberry Lane</u> by Mary Miller

March 11th

Love & Fear

Did you know that the opposite of love is really fear? Most people think it's hate but it's not. The real enemy of love is fear. The fear to be, say, or do anything. When you are afraid, you cannot love. It's impossible because fear clouds all your emotions. It muddies your thoughts and it confuses the body. You don't know where to turn. You don't know who to trust. It's amazing when you realize the power that fear can hold over your life. The good news? I believe fear can be alleviated with knowledge. They say "knowledge is power." You don't have to embrace fear, but you shouldn't run from it either. Knowledge is like a light in a darken room. You don't have to be afraid of the dark. LIGHTS! CAMERA!! ACTION!!!

CHANDLER: Oh, Robert, why do this now?

ROBERT: I doubt I would have … if you hadn't come to me first.

CHANDLER: You could have waited.

ROBERT: I didn't know if I'd get another chance! I was afraid by morning you'd be gone.

Excerpt from the play <u>Virgin Tears</u> by Mary Miller

March 12ᵗʰ

A good cry.

Sometimes you just have to cry. Sit down and *boo hoo* with all the gusto that's in you. Because sometimes you just can't take it any longer and the only way to get it out of your system is a good old-fashioned cry. I'm not talking about those quiet, two tissue type, crying ... I'm talking about the wailing, entire box of tissue, crying. Crying that reaches deep down in your gut and shakes your whole body. A good cry is good for the soul. It rids the heart of all the muck and mire that has accumulated over time. We like to think of ourselves as strong. We picture crying as a weakness. But it's a strength to be able to cry, because life, like a Shakespearean play, can be one tragedy after another. Give yourself permission to have a good cry ... so you can laugh again later.

WOMAN: Come here, Child. What you need is a good cry. That's all that's ailing you.

CHILD: (fighting back the tears) I don't want to cry.

WOMAN: You gots to cry. Cry 'til all the pain inside you is washed away. Then you'll cry a little more. I know.

Excerpt from the play Take Proper Care by Mary Miller

March 13th

Family ties.

Family! You can't live with 'em and you can't live without 'em. Family is family and we all have one! Sometimes the only thing you have in common with each other is the fact that you happen to be: sisters, brothers, mothers, fathers, cousins, aunts, uncles etc! Your family is your family ... but not all families are related. The definition for me of a *real* family is the person who is willing to go that extra mile for me when I need it most. The person I can call at 3:00 a.m. who won't hang up the phone! We all are born into a family and we have no choice in that decision. Some families are large. Some are small. Some are close and others only get together on special occasions and holidays. We may not have the chance to choose our family but we all have the chance to choose our friends ... choose well and they become the family ties that bind.

ALLISON: You're not going to lose that.

LOUISE: I feel it slipping away right now. As much as I love my family and I do ... the book club makes me feel bold, sassy, arrogant. Like I did in college.

FRAN: Those were brilliant days.

Excerpt from the play Waiting for Oprah by Mary Miller

March 14ᵗʰ

Smile first.

They could be the words to a Country Western song: "if you want to be happy *smile first* ... if you want people to like you *smile first* ... if you want to look your best *smile first.*" Smile first is the simplest, easiest, most cost effective thing you can do to win friends and influence people. Because when you smile first you win! No matter what game you're playing. No matter how high the stakes. No matter who is involved. A smile is both disarming and charming! Make it a point to always smile first and get ready to take center stage. You're about to win more friends and influence more people than you've ever dreamed possible.

CHANDLER: *(flirting, she smiles and waves)*   Hey Bobby ... *remember me?*

ROBERT: *(pleased) Chandler?! Well, I'll be damned. I didn't see you standing there. Come here.*

(He smiles. She goes to him, he hugs her and she hugs him back)

Excerpt from the play <u>Virgin Tears</u> by Mary Miller

March 15th

Better late than never.

Some days just get away from you. You wake up with every good intention of accomplishing all your goals and then life happens. On those days the best thing you can do is give yourself a little breathing room. Let go of your expectations and be still. Sometimes answers come to us when we least expect them. Most of the time they don't come with a trumpet roar or a cannon blast! They come in those rare moments when all the voices in our head finally quiet down and we can actually hear ourselves think. Those quiet moments when we have all but given up hope. That's when inspiration hits ... and it's always better late than never.

JACKSON: No harm in thinking. No harm in dreaming.

RUTH: (frightened) Oh Lord, it's been so long. I didn't know I could feel this way again. I killed off hope inside of me a long time ago. (pause) It scares me now to think if might be real.

JACKSON: Ain't nothing to be scared of.

Excerpt from the play I Witness by Mary Miller

March 16th

Day by day.

The best way I know to get through life is one day at a time ... day by day. When I was an actress in New York I used to learn my lines a paragraph at a time, day by day, until I got them all down. For the really big scripts I'd take them a page at a time, because looking at the whole script could overwhelm me. As a writer it's the same only in reverse! I start with a word and I write every day and by the end of the week, if I'm lucky, I'll have a paragraph worth saving. But I don't know that when I start. I just start with one word and follow that with another and then another and another. Life is like that. You don't know what you will get but if you take it one day at a time you'll enjoy what you have ... day after day.

MIA: You know my Momma got sober once ... for almost a year when I was fourteen ... but she couldn't take it one day at a time. She kept looking at the big picture. Sometimes the big picture is too much to look at and still hold on.

JANICE: (understanding) I try to look at as little of it as possible.

Excerpt from the play <u>Waiting for Oprah</u> by Mary Miller

March 17th

The gap in between.

Stress is the gap between where you are and where you want to be. Nothing more. Nothing less. If you think of stress in terms of a physical gap it's easier, in my mind, to close it. You know where you are, that is your starting point. You know where you want to be, that is your end point. How fast you get from A to B is the degree to which you have stress in your life. It makes sense ... doesn't it? When you plot the points out in a straight line you can begin to see the solution. It's simply a matter of focus. Think of life like a game of chess. The best chess players envision the end of the game before they start. With every move they make, they're following a predetermined strategy in their mind to win. Those of us who go from pillar to post waste not only energy but time. Focus on where you are ... envision where you want to be ... and begin to fill the gap in between.

(Suddenly they both jerk forward in their seats ... and stop still.)

DORIE: Oh my God? What happened?

JOHN: Looks like we stopped.

DORIE: Why?

JOHN: We seem to be stuck.

Excerpt from the play <u>Ferris Wheel</u> by Mary Miller

March 18th

The physical act of writing.

There is something different that happens in the brain when you physically write a word as opposed to typing and texting ... and that is the physical connection between your body and your mind. A connection a computer can only mimic. The physical act of writing is more intense, more intimate, and more immediate. The physical act of writing makes whatever you write real. Real joy. Real pain. Real anger. Real love. To actually *feel* the word as you write it makes you more aware of what you are saying and gives it a life of it's own. Give yourself time to actually write your thoughts down. Pick up a pen and paper and discover what you really think.

ADULT CHILD: (V.O.) August 12, 1955. I remember. I kept a five-year diary that year. It was a birthday present I opened early ... two months before I turned ten. In 1955 Eddie Fisher married Debbie Reynolds. Rosa Parks refused to ride in the back of the bus and Bill Haley and the Comets sang "Rock Around the Clock". We shared a lot of things that year, she and I. Nehi Sodas, Moonpies, Davy Crockett "Coonskin" caps, the Mickey Mouse Club ... and the death of my parents.

Excerpt from the play <u>Take Proper Care</u> by Mary Miller

March 19th

The art of perfection.

To be perfect at anything you first have to be good. To be good at anything you first have to start. Most people never get to where they want to go ... because they never get started in the first place! You know who I'm talking about. They're always "fixing" to do something some time, but never get around to doing anything any time. The problem when you strive for perfection with the first shot out of the gate is that it isn't going to happen. No matter how much you want it. No how much you need it. Perfection doesn't happen the first time out. Perfection comes with years and years of trying to be good. So don't let your quest for perfection stop you from being good ... and maybe even great.

DOWNSTAIRS: The last time anybody attempted doing something as stupid as this was in 1986! Don't you think if it was worth doing -- somebody would have done it before now?!?

UPSTAIRS: People were too busy making money before to worry about the Guinness Book of World Records.

DOWNSTAIRS: Exactly

UPSTAIRS: Times are tighter now. People read more.

Excerpt from the play At 3:00 O'clock in the Morning by Mary Miller

March 20th

DNA

Is our DNA working against us? Now I don't know much about DNA except what I learned in High School science, which wasn't much. But it was enough to make me aware that there are forces in my body that might be working against my being happy. Fact: DNA is designed to continue the species - the human species. Fact: The human species does best when it is challenged. Fact: When we are challenged we become our most creative self. But challenges do not make us happy. We as individuals are happiest most of the time, when things are running smoothly. We work to be comfortable so we can enjoy the life around us ... and we don't want anything to change! But internally our body may be working against us. Our DNA makes us worry, fret, stress, and complain because our DNA is always looking for a better way. Unfortunately the "better way" is often the more stressful way ... by its very nature. We would never have invented the light bulb if we had been content to stay in the dark. Once the light bulb had been invented we increased our time to worry by 100%. But when the power goes out I doubt there's anyone out there who wants to return to the days without electricity. So don't blame yourself if you worry, blame your DNA! Turn on the light, write a complicated play, and embrace a life of change.

LOUISE: When Oprah comes it's going to change everything.

ALLISON: Louise what do you expect is going to happen?

LOUISE: Something wonderful. Oprah is the epitome of everything good.

Excerpt from the play <u>Waiting for Oprah</u> by Mary Miller

March 21st

Spring Cleaning

Spring is the time of year when we really get aggressive with cleaning out our house, our closets, and our mind. The long cold winter is behind us (for the most part!) and sunny days are ahead. Spring is the season of endless possibilities, because spring is the season of birth and renewal. It is fitting that we take a moment to throw out the old and welcome the new. In the theater this was the time we repainted the stage, repaired the fixtures, restored the costumes, and reinvigorated the ensemble. Spring cleaning is not just a ritual that marks the end of winter ... it's the one time of the year that we actually throw away things that we don't need any more in order to make room for something new. Make room for something new in your life ... do a little spring cleaning today.

ADELE: I could use your help.

CHANDLER: My help doing what?

ADELE: Cleaning house. I was thinking of going through it and throwing everything away. Starting over.   It's an old house but it wasn't always such a bad place to live, was it?

Excerpt from the play <u>Virgin Tears</u> by Mary Miller

March 22nd

Chinese stress test.

It is said that the Chinese word for crisis is written by combining the symbols for the words *danger* and *opportunity*. Most of us want to avoid a crisis in our lives ... and only a fool would create one. But when confronted with a crisis it can be comforting to think, in the middle of a dangerous situation, there lies a golden opportunity. Almost all amazing success stories were born out of failures. You can read story after story about people being fired and forming their own companies and rising to the top. Or the featured star falling and the understudy going on stage. It's almost a cliché because it's so true. So what is a Chinese stress test? It's simply surviving the crisis because in the end the one who survives thrives.

BERNICE: You're still dead, aren't you.

CLARICE: (quietly) Yes. Three months, two weeks, one or two days...

BERNICE: ... give or take a few hours. But who's counting?

(They look at one another in silence. It should be obvious that the both have been counting.)

Excerpt from the play <u>Mulberry Lane</u> by Mary Miller

March 23rd

Owning the role.

It's your life own it! Step up to the plate and take responsibility for the part you are playing. Realize that the things that happen are a result of what you have done. You are not a bystander. Life doesn't just happen it evolves, whether you mean for it to or not. Theater is a living-breathing thing. That's what makes it exciting. That's what makes it unique night after night. Life is a living-breathing thing too. That's what makes it exciting. If you are not excited about your life, figure out why. If your heart is not truly committed to the part you are playing the audience will notice. The critic will pan you. So, how do you know if the role you're playing is right for you? Ask yourself do you want to play it night after night and twice on Wednesday (matinee!) It's your part to play ... why not own the role.

CLARICE: Bernice, if you had given one ounce of that energy to yourself—you could have done anything you ever wanted!!

BERNICE: I did what I wanted. I am doing what I want.

Excerpt from the play <u>Mulberry Lane</u> by Mary Miller

March 24th

Best-case scenario.

I have a friend who always says: "I like to think of the worst-case scenario so that when it's not as bad I'm relieved." I understand the concept but I respectfully disagree. When you spend your time thinking of the worst-case scenario ... often times the worst case materializes. And even when it doesn't ... when you think of the worst-case scenario you actually put your body through the emotions. Physically it takes a toll on your body whether it happens or not! Why do that? The better way, in my opinion, is to focus on the best-case scenario. Play out all the best possible solutions in your mind ... and put those ideas into practice. If you play out the best-case scenario in your mind, chances are the best-case scenario may play out in your life!

CLARICE: *You're going to be wonderful.*

BERNICE: *(unsure) I don't know. What if I can't remember lines?*

CLARICE: *You've never forgotten anything in your life.*

BERNICE: *What if they don't like me?*

CLARICE: *What's not to like.*

BERNICE: *What if I get scared?*

CLARICE: *You're too old to get scared.*

Excerpt from the play Mulberry Lane by Mary Miller

March 25th

Walk away.

Sometimes you just have to walk away. Sometimes you just have to leave. You weigh all the options and the only one that makes sense is to move on. Life is like that. Things happen, feelings get hurt, things get said. Sometimes you have a bad day. Sometimes you have more than one bad day. When you are having more bad days than good days ... it's time to think about walking away. Life is short and you owe it to yourself. No play runs forever. Even the longest running show has its last performance. Its final curtain call. Sometimes we just come to the end of a run for no particular reason ... it's just time to bring down the lights and go home. The wonderful thing about theatre is the stage never stays dark for long. There is always a new show waiting in the wings that is eager and excited to take the stage once again. Don't be afraid to walk away ... one show's ending is another show's beginning.

ALLISON: Fran? Do you really think George means for you to kill him when it gets too bad?

FRAN: No. I think he means it's OK for me to let him go.

Excerpt from the play <u>Waiting for Oprah</u> by Mary Miller

March 26th

End of the World

There is a panic that sets in when you become afraid and it can become irrational. It's why I never like to give or get bad news at night. It's always worse in the dark. In the dark our imagination can run away from us. We can actually picture the end of the world in the dark. But on a beautiful sunny day the end of the world rarely crosses our minds. People have been prophesying about the literal end of the world since the beginning of time. When I was in college the cry was "repent now the end is near." But it wasn't. And it isn't. And yet, it can feel like the end of the world when you experience a loss. You can wish it was the end of the world, but when the world doesn't end, the thing you begin to realize is that you can have a good day. Not every day. Not two days in a row. But you can have a good day every now and then ... and you can let the memory of that good day carry on to the next and the next and the next. Because it is not the end of the world, today or tomorrow.

BERNICE: *(sincerely) I miss you.*

CLARICE: *(smiling) You barely tolerated me when I was alive; don't give me this missing crap.*

BERNICE: *You really should watch your language Clarice ... when I get to heaven I'm going to give you hell!*

CLARICE: *(sincerely) I'm counting on it.*

Excerpt from the play <u>Mulberry Lane</u> by Mary Miller

March 27th

Making Happiness

In the world of wellness, they say, you don't find happiness you make it. The question is ... who are they? ... and how do you make anything? ... much less happiness. It's these kinds of platitudes that give wellness a bad name! Because they make it sound easy ... when it's not. Making happiness is the hardest work you will ever do, if you're willing to try. Making happiness demands a 24/7 vigil that few of us have the strength to devote our lives to. Happiness is a state of being we envy in others. If people are too happy we call them naive or innocent (as if there's something wrong with that!) But I believe it is the true sage among us who understands happiness. They know its value, its strength, and its pain. Some say we stumble on happiness, walking down the yellow-brick road gathering daisies along the way.   But that's happiness in the movies and once they "find" happiness in a movie that's the end of the show. The lights come up and the actors take a bow ... as if they have solved a major problem and the rest is easy. In reality, once you've found happiness, that's when the real work begins. Now it's time to roll up your sleeves put on your hard hat and try to make it happen for you again day after day.

CHANDLER: *And you're happy?*

ROBERT: *Yes.*

Excerpt from the play <u>Virgin Tears</u> by Mary Miller

March 28th

Breathe

When all else fails, breathe! It's good advice because it works. Often times when we are our most stressed-out it's because we haven't taken time to breathe. Years ago that "breathing time" was called a cigarette break. People who smoked actually were allowed to take a break from their work to go smoke a cigarette. It wasn't the best time for our health … but it probably did help save many careers. The thing about it was during that break people would actually get up from their desk and go breathe. Yes, I know they were breathing in toxic air … but this is not about the dangers of smoking it's about the need to breathe. I once quipped because I didn't smoke that I was going to take a break to breathe. Everyone thought I was joking … but it was probably the best idea I've ever had. Of course, I didn't do it then but I do it now! Try it. Go take a break to breathe. You may come back with a totally different perspective on life and work.

DORIE: Oh God. What if they make us climb out on a ladder?! (panic) I can't climb out on a ladder. I'm going to be sick.

JOHN: Just take a deep breath. It's mind over matter. Just breathe. Breathe.

(They both breathe together, she a deep breath and he like he's smoking an imaginary cigarette.)

Excerpt from the play <u>Ferris Wheel</u> by Mary Miller

March 29th

Dance like nobody's watching.

During my days as a performer in New York I looked like the perfect Song & Dance persona ... when in reality I couldn't carry a note in a bucket and I still have two left feet. But that doesn't mean that when I'm alone I don't dance around the house in my bare-feet; tap dancing to music I only hear in my head. Those are the best days. Because I truly am dancing like nobody's watching ... because nobody is watching, not even me! I remember my first experience in a formal dance class ... the thing that intimidated me the most was the great big floor-to-ceiling mirror. I couldn't look at myself and dance too, so I quit. Mind you, I've never quit dancing; I just quit looking at myself trying to do it!

CHANDLER: Do you ever dance anymore, Mattie? Just put on a record and dance? (Chandler stands and starts to hum) Come on.

MATTIE: I can't dance.

CHANDLER: Come on. Like we did as kids on Daddy's feet. Come stand on mine and we'll dance around the house.

Excerpt from the play <u>Virgin Tears</u> by Mary Miller

March 30ᵗʰ

One potato two potato…

Remember when we were kids, this was how we picked sides for a team. One potato, two potato, three potato, four. We all put our fist in and the leader would count off. Five potato, six potato, seven potato, more! The person singled out when you reached the word "more" would be relegated to the right or left side of the room. We'd go through this process until everyone had been touched and the teams were chosen. It was fair and it was fun. I don't remember anyone ever crying over … one potato two potato … not like they did when two leaders were selected and they went about choosing sides by picking those from the best to the worst. Songs have been written about those chosen last. It's a lesson we could learn again, because … one potato two potato … gives us an opportunity to discover something about others that we would never have learned if we were all simply chosen by what other people thought we did best.

DOWNSTAIRS: But it will be broken. Whatever you do. They'll revise it. It won't last forever. If you can do it, someone else is bound to be able to do it better … longer … quicker … than you!

UPSTAIRS: You don't know that. You don't know me. You don't know anything about me.

Excerpt from the play <u>At 3:00 O'clock in the Morning</u> by Mary Miller

March 31st

Writing the Dialogue: Take Care

"Take care" is a common salutation that's used in everyday conversation. But as much as we hear it, do we ever act on it? How do you actively "take care"? To me it's not just about taking care of yourself, but taking care of others. Take care to be kind. Take care to be generous. Take care to be fair. "Take care" is a way of saying you love someone. Not in a sexual way but in a way that means you'd miss them if anything were to happen to them. To tell someone to "take care" when you leave them is a way of saying you want to see them again. "Take care" is a way of saying be careful ... stay out of harms way ... look both ways before crossing the street! Good advice when we were kids and even better today. Take care!

BERNICE: I'm going. I'm going. I'm going.

(As Bernice gathers her stuff to exit, Clarice suddenly calls out.)

CLARICE: Bernice! (with deep affection) Take care.

Excerpt from the play <u>Mulberry Lane</u> by Mary Miller

April 1st

Happy Birthday...April Fools

Happy Birthday to me! Happy Birthday to me! Yes, it's my birthday ... no fooling!! I was born on April Fool's Day and it's given me license to lie about my age ever since. I think that has kept me young. Because when you lie about your age, you have to act young ... and when you act young, you feel young. You do! Don't take my word for it ... pick an age ... any age. For the next 24 hours try acting that age! At the end of the day see how you feel? My bet is, you will feel younger. You may be tired. Acting young can be exhausting ... but I bet you'll feel fresher, brighter, and happier. The past is the past, but that doesn't mean you can't go back in time. Allow yourself to be any age you want to be today ... after all it's APRIL FOOLS!!

(Babs holds up a cut out "HAPPY BIRTHDAY" banner.)

LIZBETH: (reading) HAPPY BIRTHDAY. (beat) For the Baby Jesus!

BABS: No, stupid! For Mother. In exactly one hour ... she'll be sixty!

Excerpt from the play <u>A Christmas House</u> by Mary Miller

April 2nd

Health, Wealth, Happiness

Of these three states-of-being (Health, Wealth, Happiness) only one is really important. The question is which one? If you had asked me ten years ago I would have said health ... because my health was bad. I was diagnosed with cancer and would have given anything for better health. When I lived in New York I would have given anything for more wealth. I still would give just about anything for more wealth. But if I had a choice and I had to choose ... happiness would be the state-of-being I would choose. Without happiness ... health and wealth don't add up to much. So, if you know what it feels like to be happy ... hold on to that feeling. It's the best state-of-being in the world.

MIA: You know what we should do? We should read a good old-fashioned romance novel.

ALLISON: I am not reading a book with a character named Rafael.

JANICE: Where do they come up with those names? I've never met anyone named: Yardley or Armando.

LOUISE: Mia's right. We should pick a romance. One with a happy ending.

Excerpt from the play Waiting for Oprah by Mary Miller

April 3rd

Hope

It may be irrational but 'hope' makes a difference. The scientists are always trying to prove scientifically that there is no such thing as 'hope' and that there is no real difference between those who are optimistic and those who are pessimistic. But the problem is, there is a difference, and it shows up time and time again. The brain reacts differently when you think positively. If you think you are smarter, you act smarter. If you think you are healthier, you stay healthy. (And even when you get sick, your optimism helps the healing process.) If you think you are happy, you are happy. It doesn't mean that you don't hope for more ... you can always strive for more that keeps us upright and moving forward. But to hope for a better future and act on it is the key to success anywhere! Even the scientists will agree with that!

L.E.: Merrillee, you are coming home with me. Right now!

MERRILLEE: No, I can't. I am going with the light!

L.E.: But what if it doesn't come!

MERRILLEE: It is coming. It has to come! Now stop thinking negative thoughts, Lenora Elaine, you've got to stop it ... please.

Excerpt from the play <u>Light Burgers</u> by Mary Miller

April 4th

Unfinished Dreams

We all have them ... *unfinished dreams* ... those dreams we had when we were children that have slipped to the back burner ... or fallen off the stove entirely! One of my favorite movies is "Sliding Doors." In it a young Gwyneth Paltrow plays a British girl who happens to miss the train to work one morning. Or at least you think she missed the train. As it turns out part of her misses the train ... the other part catches the train. As the movie plays out we watch as she lives her life, both lives, in a parallel universe. It's amazing to see because one part of her lives out her dream and the other part does not. Of course eventually the two parts come together (as they have to in reality!) but I won't spoil the movie; except to say that if you have an unfinished dream try imagining what your life would be like if you finished it. Then get busy! It's never too late to be what you wanted to be when you grew up.

When Fred first told Abigail about his plans, she was reluctant to agree. He was a strong man and had been a fine architect, but he was sixty-eight years old at the time, entirely too old to start building again she thought. And even though it had been his dream for as long as she could remember, it never occurred to her that when he bought the land he would build the house.

Excerpt from the book <u>A Christmas House</u> by Mary Miller

April 5ᵗʰ

Rewriting the script.

As a writer, the most important part of the writing process is rewriting! It can be frustrating and time consuming but unless you are willing to rewrite you will never become the writer you want to be. As much as I like to think my first thought is brilliant, it usually isn't. It's a good starting point, and it can set the pace and the tone for what is to come. But if it's your first attempt, save it, and do yourself a favor and try to write it again and make it better. For me, having that first draft under my belt is a grounding exercise. I know I have something. I know it can be better. And I know that rewriting will be worth the effort because I've done it before! The hardest thing for me (or anyone) is staring at a blank sheet of paper ... so let your imagination run wild on your first draft ... and then work on making it better by being willing to do rewrites again and again!

CHANDLER: When Daddy died I inherited a box labeled "WRITINGS". They gave it to me because I was the writer in the family. In it was everything he'd ever written. When I was little I used to watch him write. He'd come home from work, set up the card table, pull out his three ring binder and work on his novel. I can still hear his pen scratching across the page.

Excerpt from the play <u>Virgin Tears</u> by Mary Miller

April 6th

All's well that ends well!

It's done, it's over, and it's good. Shakespeare knew best! *All's well that ends well* means that even though you may have gone through hell, if whatever you did came out at all well, then maybe the hell was worth it! Sometimes when we are in the middle of a problem the only way out is to keep moving forward. But by moving forward without giving in to negativity and depression things do work out, because eventually everything comes to and end. And often in looking back from the vantage point of the end ... the journey seems worthwhile. I have a friend who once said: "I wouldn't give a million dollars for the trip but I wouldn't take a million dollars to do it again!" All's well that ends well. Wait for the end and then review the journey.

WOMAN: I didn't steal it. It was mine. I saw it hanging there.

MAN: And you took it.

WOMAN: I took it back.

(She puts her arm around his waist and they exit together back towards the funeral parlor.)

Excerpt from the play <u>Patterson's</u> by Mary Miller

April 7th

Standing Ovation

There is a reason that a standing ovation is the highest accolade you can give a production, because to get people out of their seats takes a monumental effort! Especially these days!! That's what I think theatre does best…it galvanizes people to action. Theatre has the power to communicate various points of view. When you can sit in the dark and watch actors perform in front of you, you have the opportunity to learn how other people live. Whether it's a play or a movie … theatre gives you the chance to explore other worlds … and for that alone I give it a standing ovation!

BERNICE: O Romeo, Romeo, wherefore art thou Romeo? Deny thy father and refuse thy name, or, if thou wilt not, be but sworn my love, and I'll no longer be a Capulet.

(Bernice is very good. Clarice bursts into applause. Bernice takes a bow.)

CLARICE: You're going to be wonderful.

Excerpt from the play Mulberry Lane by Mary Miller

April 8th

Places

Places is the last thing you hear backstage before the lights go up and the play begins. Places is the stage directors final warning telling you to take your 'place' and be ready to act. It is the moment in time, where everything stops for a minute before everything starts again. As an actor that was where I took my last breath as Mary Miller and my first breath as the character and I stayed in character until the end of the show. In life, calling *places* might be a better way to start the day. Stand for a moment, perfectly still, take a deep breath and then start the day. Before lights, camera, action … there's always places!

ADELE: Watch it!

(There is a pause. Suddenly Chandler falls back as if taken with the movement of the imaginary boat.)

CHANDLER: We're off!! Oh my God, it's beautiful.

MATTIE: It is beautiful.

Excerpt from the play <u>Virgin Tears</u> by Mary Miller

April 9th

Different Hats

We all wear different hats: wife, mother, sister, father, husband, son ... doctor, lawyer, and businessman. The list goes on and on! But under all these hats is often times the very same person ... you! That's what acting is, wearing different hats. But the thing that can get confusing, in life and on the stage, is when we wear these hats one on top of the other. Literally stacking them on our head like a clown performing a balancing act. That's when confusion sets in and tensions build. That's when we need to remember to change our hats as we move through the day. You don't necessarily want to be the mother at work nor can you expect to be the doctor at home. These are different roles and they have a different set of supporting characters. Figure out the hats you want to wear and then practice wearing them one at a time.

DORIE: But I bet your wife will be happy.

JOHN: I'm not married.

DORIE: (surprised) No?

JOHN: You?

DORIE: (embarrassed) Me?! No! No. ... But ... you? ... I assumed...

JOHN: No, divorced. Traveling Salesman ... only she couldn't take the traveling so she moved on.

Excerpt from the play Ferris Wheel by Mary Miller

April 10th

Helping Hands

Sometimes we just need help and that's when we reach out and hope there will be someone there. Whether it is a phone call or a visit, an e-mail or a letter. When we come to the end of our rope it's nice to know there are those out there who are willing to help. I call those people our *helping hands*. They could be anybody. Friends. Family. A passing stranger. But whoever they are, they can help save your life both literally and figuratively! The good thing about helping hands is that we all get to participate, because as much as we may need help from someone else, they may need help from us. So be a helping hand to someone else, you'll never know when you'll need the favor returned.

UPSTAIRS: (standing motionlessly) It won't matter. I've stopped. See! Go back downstairs. Get a good night's rest. Forget about it.

DOWNSTAIRS: (holding out a hand) Put your arm around my neck.

UPSTAIRS: I quit. I stopped. You were right. It won't count.

DOWNSTAIRS: Hush!

Excerpt from the play At 3:00 O'clock in the Morning by Mary Miller

April 11th

Surprise Surprise

I hate being surprised. That's probably a control issue I have with not wanting to be out of my element for too long. But I'm not alone. It seems the older I get the less and less I like the element of surprise. Take a surprise party for example: isn't it better to be able to think about it, plan for it, look forward to it rather than being shocked out of your mind, dressed in jeans with your hair dirty, type of surprise? I wonder about people who like to surprise you? Are they just trying to control your life too? Some surprises are fun, like what you get for Christmas. I've never been one to peak ... why? ... because it would spoil the surprise! But these days the surprise that happens most often is one of illness and loss, whether it's a job or a love one. So these days the only place I like to be surprised is at the theatre. And the surprise I like best ... is the one that makes me laugh!

LOUISE: I would've sworn he was dead.

FRAN: He can sit catatonic like that for hours. Sometimes his breathing is so slight even I get up to make sure he's still alive. I'm not surprised you thought he was dead. (beat) I am surprised you thought I killed him, strapped him in a seat belt, and drove over here to meet Oprah!? Louise, I'm not that crazy. Not yet.

Excerpt from the play <u>Waiting for Oprah</u> by Mary Miller

April 12th

Take the time.

Some things just take time. Usually those are the best things. Those things that we treasure the most. It's funny when you are waiting for something to happen it can seem like an eternity ... then once it happens ... it's over in a flash. I often think that time is relative in the sense that two people can experience the same time entirely differently. If you're busy it goes by fast ... if you're not it can feel like forever. But most of the time I think we rush through life. I wonder if we are so afraid to slow down that we manufacture places to go and things to do? Maybe it's time to take time and see what life is all about.

ROBERT: *Chandler, wait!*

(She stops and looks back at him. He is suddenly hesitant ... nervous ... as he takes his time and weighs his words.)

ROBERT: *Now that you mention it, there is ... something ... I'd like to ask you?*

Excerpt from the play <u>Virgin Tears</u> by Mary Miller

April 13th

The cutting room floor.

Sometimes despite our best efforts it seems everything we do ends up on the cutting room floor. How many of us, if you go all the way back to our childhood, have actually achieved our childhood dreams? In fact you don't have to go that far back. In school I remember being described as full of potential. When was the last time anyone told you that you were full of potential? I wonder what happens to that potential? I guess we get out in the real world, have to earn a living, raise a family, and a lot of things end up on the cutting room floor so to speak. Not that that's a bad place, necessarily. But I bet in everyone's life there is something that ended up on the cutting room floor that they might want to pick up and re-examine for a minute. To see if they want to add it to the final cut. After all, if you're still alive, there's still time. Then again, on second thought, you might decide that the cutting room floor is exactly where that piece of life belongs!!

WOMAN: Everything I ever wanted she took. She only wanted it because I wanted it. Then when she got it, she never cared to keep it.

MAN: Including me.

WOMAN: Especially you. But don't come running back to me now! I don't want her hand me downs.

Excerpt from the play <u>Patterson's</u> by Mary Miller

April 14ᵗʰ

Happiness is ...

For those of us who grew up with Charles Schultz "Happiness Is A Warm Puppy" especially if that puppy was Peanuts. Happiness is a thing we strive for not only in the comics but in the Constitution! The Pursuit Of Happiness is the third inalienable right just behind life and liberty. In the scheme of things, happiness is right up at the top. But how does one become happy? There are those external things like new cars, clothes, TV, i-anything! There are those internal things like good health, good friends, and good times. The search for happiness can span a lifetime of living. But to me, true happiness is just being content with oneself. That's happiness inside and out.

WOMAN: Happy I been happy to do what I do for as long as I have. The Lord's been good to me and my family.

Excerpt from the play Take Proper Care by Mary Miller

April 15th

Tax time!

Suddenly it's crunch time. Time to pay the government what you owe them. Taxes for me are a chance to look back over the past year and see exactly where my money went? It's the only time I get excited about spending a lot of money on my career ... because if my accountant works it right, I can get some of the money back! But the main thing that happens to me at this time of the year is a reassessing of where I've been and where I'm going.

CLARICE: You've got old clothes, old magazines, old bills, old movie receipts. Who ever heard of saving old movie receipts?

BERNICE: They are for tax purposes.

CLARICE: Tax Purposes!? Tax purposes my foot! They were yours and George's and you can't bring yourself to throw them out!

Excerpt from the play Mulberry Lane by Mary Miller

April 16th

Bless your heart...

Southern expressions are one of a kind ... we say what we mean, but, what we say doesn't always reflect exactly what we are thinking. In fact sometimes it can be exactly the opposite, which can be confusing to our Northern friends. Take the expression *'bless your heart'* when you hear these words, directed at you, you better get ready to run because something bad is coming your way! It's either going to be condescending, mean, or down right catty ... all disguised under the heading of a blessing. The expression itself is most frequently use in reference to someone's brains or beauty; as in *bless her heart* she's so dumb... or *bless his heart* he's so ugly! It's fun to write as dialogue and even more to say on stage ... but trust me, in life, you don't ever want anyone to bless your heart!

CLARICE: Well, bless his heart! Who would have thought George was gay!

BERNICE: (defensive) Gay?! He most certainly was not!

CLARICE: I always liked George! I was rooting for George.

Excerpt from the play <u>Mulberry Lane</u> by Mary Miller

April 17ᵗʰ

Dr. Wilson! Dr. Wilson!!

These were the first words I ever said on camera. I was playing the part of a nurse on the soap opera *The Guiding Light* and a tractor trailer truck had jack-knifed on the highway and now Dr. Wilson, the new good looking young intern at Cedars Hospital, was needed to perform brain surgery! It was a very dramatic moment. I answered the phone, took the message, and yelled for the doctor as they wheeled the patient into the operating room. Of course at the end of the scene the director (from his hidden booth overlooking the stage) noticed that our patient was still wearing her boots (did I mention how cold it was on those shooting stages?) and the scene had to be re-shot. We did it a total of five times before we got the boots off and the name of the disease pronounced correctly. That was the start of my career. So you don't have to worry, you are in good hands. I may not be a doctor, but I have played a nurse on TV.

NURSE #1: Dr. Wilson! Dr. Wilson!! You're wanted in surgery...

Exert from the soap opera THE GUIDING LIGHT performed by Mary Miller

April 18th

Lost and Found

If you've ever lost something, and I'm sure everyone has, you know the sickening feeling of loss. You wrack your brain for where you may have put it last. You look, time and time again, in the same logical spot to no avail. Then you start looking in places you never were ... just on the off chance that it may have actually sprouted legs and walked away. Then in a final last ditch attempt you begin to look in places where it never should be ... like the refrigerator or freezer! The places an Alzheimer patient may have put it. Sometimes there's actually a sense of relief when it's not there. But lost is loss and until you can relax and take a deep breath, sometimes what you are looking for ends up being right in front of you.

ALLISON: Fran when was the first time you noticed something was seriously wrong with George?

FRAN: When I found his shoes in the refrigerator, sitting between the pickles and a left-over casserole.   I thought he was drinking.

MIA: Maybe he was.

FRAN: No, they weren't randomly tossed in the fridge. They were carefully placed side-by-side as if that were the perfect place to put shoes. And I was the one foolish for questioning it, standing there wondering where his socks were.

Excerpt from the play <u>Waiting for Oprah</u> by Mary Miller

April 19ᵗʰ

Celebrating little things.

Have you ever said this: "When I become _____(fill in the blank) I'm really going to celebrate!" And so often the thing you had planned to celebrate either never happens or when it does you neglect to celebrate it? We miss so many opportunities to celebrate by waiting for something big enough to merit a celebration that, often, we never celebrate anything at all. Celebrate something today. I don't know what that something will be ... that's up to you. They say life is a celebration, but you have to be the one to throw the party! Don't put off the party any longer waiting for something special ... celebrate little things in your life. They may turn out to be bigger than you think.

MERRILLEE: *We ought to throw a party for Mason. You know, tie in his return with the coming of the light and have a theme party.*

L.E.: *Merrillee after what's happened to Frank, I doubt anybody is interested in a party right now.*

MERRILLEE: *People are always interested in a party. It helps during agonizing times. (pause) And we haven't had a big theme party around here with costumes and party favors in a long time.*

Excerpt from the play Light Burgers by Mary Miller

April 20ᵗʰ

Compassion

Compassion may just be the greatest emotion on earth. It is greater than love because love sometimes fades. It's greater than empathy because it takes more of a commitment. Greater than hope because it is encompasses hope and so much more. Compassion is actually being able to put yourself, your whole self, in the shoes of another person. To see as they see, feel as they feel, think as they think. If you have compassion for someone else, you can't hurt them, you can't cheat them, you can't be anything but kind. Compassion is the one emotion that can truly change the world.

UPSTAIRS: You should have just bought some earplugs.

DOWNSTAIRS: I can't sleep with earplugs.

(They look at one another. There is a moment of recognition between the two of them.)

DOWNSTAIR: (CONT.) I can't sleep either.

Excerpt from the play At 3:00 O'clock in the Morning by Mary Miller

April 21ˢᵗ

Magic

I believe in magic. It's almost a prerequisite to being in theatre, because nowhere else on earth is magic more prevalent than on the stage. Actors experience it every night when they transform their lives and become totally different people. The audience anticipates it sitting in the dark; waiting for something to excite them, inspire them, transport them, and thrill them. Because that's what theatre can do ... and if that's not magic, then I don't know what magic is!

(Frank "pulls" a quarter out of L.E.'s ear and holds it out to her but she does not take it.)

L.E.: (gently, pushing him away) Stop it.

FRANK: It's magic L.E.

L.E.: You don't believe in magic.

FRANK: I'd like to believe in magic, and UFO's, and flying saucers, and life on Mars, and Heaven ... where old friends meet.

Excerpt from the play Light Burgers by Mary Miller

April 22nd

Selling the part.

I have now come to the conclusion that the best acting is not really acting but selling the part. The best actor is a great salesman, because in order to sell anything you have to come at it with conviction and enthusiasm as if it were the most important thing in the world both on stage and in life. They say, a good salesman can sell anything, and sometimes that takes on a negative connotation because sometimes what they are selling is not something you want to buy. But in the world of theatre the audience is anxious to buy what a good actor is selling. We go to a play or movie hoping to believe. We sit in the dark waiting to be sold. We have our money out ready to buy. All you have to do is sell them the part.

BERNICE: *Acting was your dream not mine!*

CLARICE: *That's a bold face lie! You take it back!! I only wanted to be an actress so I could be like you.*

Excerpt from the play <u>Mulberry Lane</u> by Mary Miller

April 23rd

A One Woman Show

How often have you thought that what you do is a one woman show? You clean, you cook, you go to work, you take care of the kids, and look after one another. A woman's job is never done, and yet, more often than not, we rarely tire, we hardly complain, and most of the time we laugh. But the one thing we need to remember in the midst of this performance is to take a moment to take care of ourselves. Take time to pat yourself on the back for the job you do ... whether it's at home or in the office ... it's important to recognize yourself as the amazing performer you are and give yourself a round of applause.

DOWNSTAIRS: I'll have you know my hands touch over two million dollars a day. Individually handling every bill that comes in and goes out. Crossing my palms. (opening both hands in a show of frustration) For twenty-five years I've worked with people who are so rude it's hard to imagine that they can actually walk away from me and trust that I will put their money in the bank.

Excerpt from the play <u>At 3:00 O'clock in the Morning</u> by Mary Miller

April 24th

Waiting Time

I am good at a lot of things but I'm terrible at waiting. In my opinion, waiting is one of the hardest things we ever have to do. It can be one of the most stressful times in life, because when we are waiting we suspend our normal every day life and stop everything; for however long it takes, to get an answer. Funny thing is it doesn't matter how big the question is, waiting is hard. It's hard to stay positive. It's hard to continue to believe. It's hard to stay true to your dream and trust yourself. Waiting is when we are most vulnerable. It's when that house we thought we had built with brick and mortar suddenly feels as if it's nothing more than a house of cards that could tumble over at any minute. I don't know why we don't get stronger as we wait? Maybe it's because we feel powerless and nothing is more frightening than sitting in a waiting room waiting for others to determine your fate.

CHANDLER: I do have faith but not in wooden statues that cry real tears.

ADELE: You've never been here. You've never seen the people gather around, holding sick children in their arms. Waiting. Watching. Praying to catch a glimpse of something Holy.

Excerpt from the play Virgin Tears by Mary Miller

April 25th

Own your defeats.

More often than not I like to focus on victory ... but losing can be an instrumental tool in winning. We cannot win every time we step up to the plate. It's impossible. In fact, if you win every time, you've set the bar too low. (Note: I'm not an advocate for setting the bar too high either!) But there is something immeasurable about owning our loses. So often people look for excuses, figure out ways to blame something or someone else when they don't get what they want or feel they deserve. Sometimes that's true. But those characters quickly become tedious and boring on stage and in life! Sometimes you just lose the game, the part, the job, the deal, you name it! When that happens it's important to own up to it ... it's what makes us all human and enables us to grow. Because ultimately it's only by owning our loses that we can truly claim victory!!

L.E.: Why are you here?

MASON: Dillard is my home.

L.E.: New York is your home.

MASON: Home? (he laughs to himself) You know, the first day I arrived in New York City, I saw this old woman walking in the street carrying everything she owned in two plastic shopping bags saying "stop, stop" quietly over and over again to herself but she kept on going. L.E., New York is nobody's home. It let's you live there as long as you can ... once you can't it rolls right on over you.

Excerpt from the play <u>Light Burgers</u> by Mary Miller

April 26th

Tomorrow is another day!

These may be the most important four words in *Gone With The Wind*, because that is exactly what propelled that storyline for over a 1,000 pages. It's what enabled Scarlet to survive war, death, famine, and poverty. Now you may not think of Scarlet O'Hara as the perfect role model but you do have to admit she survived and thrived in a hell of a world. No matter what was happening around her... she got through it all by remembering that tomorrow is another day and you can never know what tomorrow will bring. And isn't that worth getting up for every morning, just to see what tomorrow will bring?

L.E.: (somewhat panicky) Oh Lord, this has to be postmarked no later than tomorrow to beat the Gold Seal Date and I want to make sure it gets out in the early morning mail. Otherwise I forfeit my $5 million dollars to an alternate winner!

MERRILLEE: (interjecting) I have a stamp, right in here.

Excerpt from the play <u>Light Burgers</u> by Mary Miller

April 27ᵗʰ

Best of intentions.

Sometimes the best of intentions go awry. You can mean well but what you do either doesn't work, loses money, or simply falls flat on its face. It doesn't mean that when you started you wanted anything less than the best. I sometimes think we forget this. We forget that nine times out of ten, people really do try to do the best they can; and it is with every good intention that most projects begin. How they end can be a totally different thing. But no one sets out to fail. Every writer wants to write the great American novel. Every actor at one time or another has envisioned receiving an Academy Award and if they're honest they've probably rehearsed their speech to the bathroom mirror! Not every one can win but there is honor in trying especially when you try with the best of intentions.

UPSTAIRS: Have you ever told anyone you loved 'em?

DOWNSTAIRS: (bristling) This isn't about me.

UPSTAIRS: I didn't think so.

DOWNSTAIRS: I have too. They just didn't love me back, and I stood there like a fool waiting for nothing. I swore I'd never do that again. And I haven't!

UPSTAIRS: Damn.

Excerpt from the play <u>At 3:00 O'clock in the Morning</u> by Mary Miller

April 28th

Achilles' Heel

It was born of the Greek mythology. Achilles was dipped in the river Styx by his mother to make him invincible. She held him by the heel and dipped him into the water ... making all but the heel impenetrable, which eventually led to his demise. Try as we will to protect ourselves and our loved ones, sometimes our best efforts can be our undoing. Sometimes we just have to let what happens, happen, and hope for the best. We all put up a front of invincibility but underneath we all have an Achilles' heel when you dig deep enough. And that's not a bad thing ... in fact I think it's probably what gives us our humanity.

ADELE: Do you know Daddy once bet Mr. Harris that I could walk around the lake? It was over three miles around and I was only seven years old. But I walked that lake. My feet were cut and blistered, but Daddy won the bet! He took his money and carried me home.

CHANDLER: He should have given you the money.

ADELE: (turning on Chandler)   He was a good man! He only wanted the best for us.

CHANDLER: He just never allowed anyone to fail!

Excerpt from the play <u>Virgin Tears</u> by Mary Miller

April 29th

Picture This!

One of the most important things to remember in writing is to paint the picture for the reader. It is our job as writers to make sure that the reader sees what we see, experiences what we experience, feels what we feel. That's the magic of writing to create a world on the page that the reader can see. That's what all great art is really ... creating other worlds for people to experience. Painters do it on canvas. Actors do it on the stage. Writers do it on the page. So when writing your play concentrate not only on what you say ... but everything around you. Paint the picture of the world you want to live in and start by describing it word by word.

L.E.: You look at a 'mysterious' light that talks to you in a garble language you can only understand in your sleep and you don't think to ask it a single question?!

MERRILLEE: Well, there was one question burning in the back of my mind, Lenora Elaine.

MASON: And that was...?

MERRILLEE: What to wear. (pause) After they invited me, I suddenly realized I didn't have a clue as to what to wear! Was it cold? Was it hot? Can you wear white?

Excerpt from the play Light Burgers by Mary Miller

April 30th

Know your audience.

In life as on the stage it's important to know who your audience is in order to best figure out how to play your role. We all play different characters when we are around different people. Watch anyone with a baby and see how long it takes them to dissolve into a babbling brook. Watch children with their parents both old and young alike. Think of your relationship with your co-workers and your boss. A friend or a lover. It's not that you have to change yourself to accommodate them so much as you need to be aware of what their sensibilities are in order to be better understood. Know your audience, it's simply a matter of caring more for someone else in the moment than you do for yourself.

DORIE: What did you do that for?

JOHN: I don't know ... I thought if I kissed you, you'd stop talking for a minute.

DORIE: Oh.

(She looks at him. He leans over and kisses her again.)

DORIE: I wasn't talking.

JOHN: I wanted to see if I enjoyed it as much the second time as I did the first.

Excerpt from the play <u>Ferris Wheel</u> by Mary Miller

May 1ˢᵗ

Plan ahead.

Sometimes despite all our best efforts it can be hard to keep the deadlines we set for ourselves. But I'm a firm believer that if you plan ahead you can accomplish anything. So, I make false deadlines for myself in order to keep moving forward. It's an old habit but it has served me well. The one thing I know that separates those who achieve from those who fail is the simple fact that those who achieve tend to finish the work. Whether it's writing a book, composing a song, or building a dream house. Plan ahead and give yourself a chance to succeed.

DOWNSTAIRS: You think you can walk around this apartment non-stop for six days?

UPSTAIRS: They give you time to go to the bathroom.

DOWNSTAIRS: Not much.

UPSTAIRS: It's enough.

Excerpt from the play <u>At 3:00 O'clock in the Morning</u> by Mary Miller

May 2nd

Rehearsal process.

We often hear that life is not a rehearsal ... and it's true, life is real and it's happening now. But that diminishes what a rehearsal is all about. Rehearsing is a vital part of life ... think of the times we practice what we want to say to the bathroom mirror. We take dry runs to make sure we know where we are going for that all important meeting that could change our life. Think of the sports professionals who practice everyday. After all practice is just another word for rehearsal. We practice it until we get it right ... and then we live it. Don't neglect the rehearsal process it's a key component to living your best life now.

ABIGAIL: You've built the same house. You realize that, don't you?

FRED: It's not exactly the same. It's better! It has everything you ever wanted. An attic ... and a pool ...

ABIGAIL: ... and six unfinished bedrooms ... with six unfinished bathrooms!

FRED: It was like getting a chance to live part of my life over again ... and getting it right, this time.

Excerpt from the play A Christmas House by Mary Miller

May 3rd

Memorization

The hardest part of acting is memorizing lines. Of course the more lines the bigger the part, but it can be daunting when you are looking at a page full of dialogue that you not only have to learn but have to deliver with conviction and authority. Memorization is a muscle, the more you use it the better you get. The greatest excuse in the world is 'I forgot.' Sometimes forgetting can be a blessing. But it's important to remember people, places, and things. It helps define who your are. The greatest loss with Alzheimer's disease is the loss of memories. Practice memorization … to keep your mind well tuned and sharp. Surprise someone and remember their name!!

MIA: Are you going to tell him what happened today?

FRAN: No. It just scares him and I hate to see him searching for something he can't remember.

LOUISE: Does he still want to see Oprah?

FRAN: He didn't mention it. I didn't ask. I doubt he remembers ever wanting to see her in the first place.

Excerpt from the play <u>Waiting for Oprah</u> by Mary Miller

May 4th

The Placebo Effect

It's a known fact these days that the placebo effect can be as much as 10%. That's a 10% improvement without treatment or medication. That's just the brain thinking it's getting better! Amazing!! If an actual drug or a treatment had that kind of effect it would be marketed as a miracle cure and they'd be right. So it begs the question, if we know a placebo is effective, why don't we focus more on the power of the mind to help keep us well? It seems to me if we actually encouraged and even taught the power of positive thinking we could improve our well-being by at least 10%. Isn't positive thinking the best example of how we all can live better lives by Acting Healthy?

FRANK: L.E.! Get your hands off my head.

L.E.: But you were bleeding.

FRANK: The doctors said it was just ketchup got smeared all over me when you laid me out on the counter.

L.E.: Ketchup my foot! That was blood.

GEORGE: L.E., you trying to ruin me?! If he says it's ketchup, it's ketchup!

MASON: Well, what ever it was, it's gone. And you're both damn lucky.

Excerpt from the play <u>Light Burgers</u> by Mary Miller

May 5th

Dropping the ball …

Dropping the ball is not the worst thing that can happen to you especially if that *ball* is full of negative energy. After all it takes two to fight. If someone throws negative energy towards you the worst thing you can do is catch it and throw it back. Because, guess what, that ball of trouble is going to come back at you even harder and faster! That's how arguments escalate into fights and fights into wars … both physically and mentally. So, whether you are on stage, backstage, or in the audience don't be afraid to drop the ball … or better yet, step aside and let it pass by you altogether.

UPSTAIRS: I'm just walking.

DOWNSTAIRS: Precisely! How can I complain? You're walking in your own apartment. Of course you can walk in your own apartment. But you can't keep walking around in your apartment at 3:00 o'clock in the morning!

(The upstairs neighbor ignores the comment, turns, and walks in the opposite direction. The downstairs neighbor turns and follows behind.)

DOWNSTAIRS: (CONT.) Look, I don't want to fight.

Excerpt from the play <u>At 3:00 O'clock in the Morning</u> by Mary Miller

May 6th

Patience is a virtue ... sometimes.

They say, patience is a virtue ... but you don't want to wait your life away. Sometimes you just have to step out and make a move and hope for the best! Life is always changing and if you expect it to stay the same while you're waiting, you're wasting your time. My suggestion, plan the best you can for the best ... and then act on it. Sometimes people confuse inactivity with patience. But most of the time the reason people wait too long is fear. Step out into the world, make your move; you rarely regret what you did as much as you regret what you didn't do.

MATTIE: You'll just have to wait for the right moment. Patience, you don't have any patience.

CHANDLER: No. I'm walking around with a drippy eyedropper in my pocket leaking down my leg.

MATTIE: It's not even time yet. We can't do anything until after 9:00 p.m. or Adele will be suspicious.

Excerpt from the play Virgin Tears by Mary Miller

May 7th

Supporting Characters

On stage the most important person next to the lead is the *supporting* character. They are never the prettiest, or the thinnest, and they never have as many lines, but the supporting character can save a show. They are the people who the lead turns to when they are in trouble if they've forgotten a line or a prop. The supporting character is the one who comes to their rescue. The unsung hero of the stage. In life, too, we have supporting characters who may never get the credit they deserve. A teacher, a coach, a friend. A supporting character is that person in your life who you can call when you need help and they actually come.

CHANDLER: You didn't tell her?

MATTIE: It's been almost two years, Chandler. I wasn't even sure you'd come back. I didn't want to disappoint her. She's been so disappointed before.

CHANDLER: I don't think disappointed is what she'll feel.

MATTIE: We're family. We should be together at times like this.

Excerpt from the play <u>Virgin Tears</u> by Mary Miller

May 8th

Three Act Play

Life is a lot like a three act play if you're lucky. The first act is the beginning years. The learning years. The molding years. The years you become who you hoped you might be. The second act is the realizing years. The years you realize who you are and what you have become and hopefully coupled with a sense of accomplishment and acceptance. The third act … well the third act is open for interpretation. The third act is the time in your life when everything that is expected of you is either done or not. In the third act you are free to be who you want to be again.

BERNICE: I went off again, didn't I?

CLARICE: Just for a second.

BERNICE: I've started to do that recently.

CLARICE: I know. You need something to occupy your time. You can't live in the past.

Excerpt from the play Mulberry Lane by Mary Miller

May 9th

Extraction

Sometimes things just have to come out. They were useful for a while, but they've outlived their usefulness and now it's time to pull 'em. Of course I'm talking about teeth here but think about the concept. As a writer, sometimes you just have to edit out that wonderful paragraph that woke you up in the middle of the night. Sometimes it just doesn't fit in with the rest of the story. In life too, sometimes you just have to extract yourself from a bad situation. Move on and see what life is like without him, her, them, or it. Sometimes an extraction is the only way back to health.

CHANDLER: At work I hate my job so much, I walk behind my boss and give her the finger, behind her back, when she's not looking like some unruly child.

ROBERT: It's all right.

CHANDLER: No. I have to quit my job. Do something else. Get out of there while people still think I'm worth working with, at this rate it's hard to tell who's crazier. Me or my boss.

Excerpt from the play <u>Virgin Tears</u> by Mary Miller

May 10th

Build a bridge.

Sometimes if you want to get from point A to point B you just have to build a bridge. Sometimes there is no easy way to get from where you are to where you want to be ... without getting your hands dirty and your feet wet. Building a bridge takes time, planning, persistence, and hard work. But it's the best hard work you'll ever do. Don't limit yourself to just building a new bridge ... maybe it's time to think about re-building those old bridges you may have burned down in the past. After all a good bridge can be a link from the past to the present and into the future. Build yourself a bridge ... it's the best way I know to get you where you want to go.

L.E.: (yelling down to him) What are you going to do with a hose?

GEORGE: I'm going to fill in that ditch so it's clear just where my property begins and the city's ends!

MASON: You aren't going to do anything but make it harder for those people who want to eat here to get here.

GEORGE: They can come through. Those that want to.

Excerpt from the play <u>Light Burgers</u> by Mary Miller

May 11th

Happy Mother's Day

Whether you are a mother or not, you've probably influenced someone's life more than you know. Whether you are a mother or not, you've probably worried about others more than you care to admit. Whether you are a mother or not, you've probably help carry the weight of the world on your shoulders. Whether you are a mother or not you are important to someone. This Mother's Day (whatever day it happens to be!) thank someone who has made a difference in your life ... whether they are a mother or not.

ABIGAIL: Watch your step. Be careful. Oh, I can't look.

LIZBETH: Momma, I'm a grown woman. You don't have to worry about me.

ABIGAIL: A grown woman my foot. You are my baby and you'll always be my baby, and as long as you are under my roof ... (she looks up) ... which is the only thing this house seems to have, I'm going to worry.

Excerpt from the play <u>A Christmas House</u> by Mary Miller

May 12th

Five Years

There is a little book I saw the other day called *5: Five*. The subtitle was: *Where Will You Be In Five Years*. A part of me started to look through it … but then a part of me stopped. It's really impossible to determine where you'll be in five years once you get past the age of twenty-five! Life sometimes takes on a life of it's own and moves us in directions we could never foresee. Sometimes they are the best of times and sometimes they are the worst. It's important to look ahead … but it's equally important to take note of the moment and enjoy it for what it is.

FRAN: How long has it been, Allison?

ALLISON: Five years next week. Can you believe it? I have my last six-month check up on Wednesday. If everything is clean … then I can go back to yearly exams like everybody else.

MIA: We should have a party and celebrate!

ALLISON: No. That's OK. I'd rather not. I'm sort of superstitious about the date. I don't want to jinx anything.

Excerpt from the play <u>Waiting for Oprah</u> by Mary Miller

May 13ᵗʰ

You saved my life!

Now that's not something you hear much as a playwright, but it happens, and it's happened to me. My play NEXT about four women waiting to get a mammogram saved the life of a friend of mine. Those are her words – not mine! She told me, after seeing the play, she went and got a mammogram and they found a lump. To this day, she credits NEXT with having saved her life. Now not every play you see is going to save your life, but it could. Theatre can hold a mirror to life and if you have the courage to look, it can change your life. I know it changed mine.

JOAN: I'm terrified.

BARBARA: Don't be. It's nothing. They put your breast in this machine and press it ... until you'll confess to anything. Your age. Your weight. Your hair color. You'd tell 'em anything they want to know and then they take a picture.

Excerpt from the play <u>NEXT</u> by Mary Miller

May 14th

Act like a dog.

Now most people will agree that man's best friend is a dog. That's because a dog is always glad to see you and they love you unconditionally without judgment or reservations!! What more could a person want in a best friend? Isn't it funny we know what we want, but we're so careful not to give it away? A dog gives his love freely. Maybe if we tried to act more like a dog, we'd learn how to love one another a little more.

JANICE: I don't want to end up alone. I'm not much of a cat person.

Excerpt from the play <u>Waiting for Oprah</u> by Mary Miller

May 15th

Sense of Smell

The sense of smell is the most overlooked and forgotten of all our five senses. And yet, it's very important to our health and wellbeing. Of course, it's nearly impossible to incorporate the sense of smell into theatre or the movies. But in life the aroma of something pleasant can release endorphins that can enhance your whole day, change your mood, and brighten your outlook. Today, go out of your way to smell something nice. Put on a little perfume in the morning. We only have five senses, it's time to exercise the sense of smell … it might save your life!

CHANDLER: Adele? Adele! Do I smell something burning?

Excerpt from the play <u>Virgin Tears</u> by Mary Miller

May 16th

It takes two.

It takes two to do just about anything. It's almost in our DNA the need for another person. Even in solitary confinement a person will find something to befriend in order to stay sane. The strangest moment in any film I've ever seen that personifies this phenomenon is the movie *Castaway* with Tom Hanks where he befriends a Wilson soccer ball and almost loses his mind when he thinks the 'ball' is lost. We in the audience are fearful as well. So if you find that you are always doing things alone, broaden your horizons and invite a friend along. It takes two to share a moment.

JOHN: Excuse me. Excuse me? I hope I'm not ... crowding you...

DORIE: (flustered/embarrassed) No.

(He slides into the empty seat next to her and takes hold to the "bar".)

Excerpt from the play Ferris Wheel by Mary Miller

May 17th

Stand up for yourself.

Sometimes you just have to stand up for yourself. You have to take a leap of faith and believe in yourself enough to stand out above the crowd. Too often we just go along to get along. Sometimes we get swept up in a crowd we don't even want to be a part of but we're afraid to be different. Being different is what makes us unique. I know as a playwright the hardest thing to do is to create a totally new and different character; and yet the real world is full of them! So when you find yourself lost in a crowd you don't want to be a part of ... stand up for yourself. You may find others following behind you.

L.E.: I thought you had seen the light.

MASON: Yeah, by myself, it's not as hard to accept the unknown by yourself. But in a crowd you start thinking what they're thinking instead of what you're thinking. Doing what they're doing. It's easy to get lost in a crowd.

Excerpt from the play <u>Light Burgers</u> by Mary Miller

May 18th

When all else fails ... smile!

A smile is the most beautiful, disarming, powerful expression we have as human beings. It can literally transform you. If you're smiling people will gravitate to you to learn the secret of your happiness. When you're smiling you release endorphins that will enhance not only your health and well-being but the health and well-being of those around you. When you're smiling you can't feel bad ... even if you are faking it. Because when you fake a smile, nobody knows it, including your body. So smile! It's a beautiful thing.

McKenzie smiled, thinking back to Lewis' casual manner in handling that potentially disastrous situation.

Excerpt from the book <u>A Matter of Grace</u> by Mary Miller

May 19ᵗʰ

Lifeline

A lifeline is a lifesaver, no matter how you look at it. It can be a physical lifeline like a rope someone throws you if you're stuck in a hole; or a metaphorical lifeline like a pep talk someone gives you when you're stuck in life. In either case a lifeline is something that actually saves your life. I know, I've thrown them and caught them. They can come from friends or family or complete strangers. Trust me you'll know one when you see it or hear it. My advice is to grab on tight and hold on!

CLARICE: Now, when you get out there treat yourself to a new outfit. Promise me you won't pull anything out of those old garbage bags!! Oh, and at the audition insist on doing a comic monologue and a serious one. Don't let 'em tell you they haven't got time. They do. And if you can't think of one yourself I've got plenty in the bottom of one of those JohnnyWalkerLiquor boxes.

Excerpt from the play <u>Mulberry Lane</u> by Mary Miller

May 20th

Respect yourself.

Do you realize the longest relationship you'll ever have with anyone ... is with yourself? Now we all know how we would like to be treated in a relationship ... with respect, love, and forgiveness. Why not take a page from that book and give it to yourself? In other words, why not practice respecting yourself. Loving yourself. Forgiving yourself. Take a look in the mirror, a good long look ... love what you like, change what you don't. You are the great love of your life ... respect yourself.

(Pearl slowly walks over to a mirror and looks at her reflection.)

PEARL: You know son. Behind this face is all the people I've ever been in my life ... and not a one of them had nothing. Still I can look at this face every day in the mirror and not have to look away. It may not be much but it's peace. Peace is about all I seem to be able to want these days.

Excerpt from the play I Witness by Mary Miller

May 21st

The Price Patrol

Some days it feels like the only solution to life's problems is for the Price Patrol to drive into your driveway and say: YOU'RE A WINNER. The problem is most days we don't play the game, buy the ticket, step up to the plate, or even go to the theatre. Sometimes you have to get off the couch to find a solution to life's problems. You have to make an effort for the Price Patrol to drive into your driveway!

L.E.: You won't catch me dragging around a suitcase waiting for an alien.

MASON: No, you're filling out a Publishers Clearing House Sweepstakes entry waiting for the Price Patrol to drive up the driveway!

Excerpt from the play <u>Light Burgers</u> by Mary Miller

May 22nd

Writing the Dialogue: What, me worry?

As a kid I loved Mad Magazine. My favorite expression was *What, me worry?* Of course back then, I didn't have much to worry about. But as time has passed, my worries have grown year after year. I suppose that's part of growing up. But the older I get now, the more I realize that expression is the true secret to life. Worry only about the things you can change and let the rest go. What, me worry? Not if I don't have to!

LOUISE: I used to worry about being vaporized now I'm afraid of being taken out by terrorists. It doesn't seem fair.

Excerpt from the play <u>Waiting for Oprah</u> by Mary Miller

May 23rd

Walking the Labyrinth

Many people think of a labyrinth as a maze or a puzzle ... but a true labyrinth is just the opposite. There's no trick to it, it just feels that way! A true labyrinth is a mirror of life. If you follow the path you will find, at times, it seems to take you further and further away from your goal. But it's only by following the path that you will eventually reach the end. You have to believe and not give up, stay the course, focus on the journey, and you will reach your goal. Trust me!

DOWNSTAIRS: (reading from the book) The first person reputed to have "walked around the world." (looking up) You're not planning on walking around the world?! That'll take years!

UPSTAIRS: No, that's the longest walk. I'm walking continually. That only took six days.

Excerpt from the play At 3:00 O'clock in the Morning by Mary Miller

May 24th

One

I've heard it said that one is a lonely number. But I don't agree. Sometimes one person is all it takes to change the world. One person to smile at you. One person to say a kind word. One person to reach out and give you a hand. One person can start a rippling effect that can be felt all over the world. One person can make a difference ... why not be that one person.

MATTIE: Please, Chandler. Just eye drop a tear. One little tear. It wouldn't be hard and it'd mean the world to Adele. I'd do it myself, but I can't. I've tried ... three times ... but every time I got close to the Virgin my hands shook so hard I didn't think they'd ever stop. That's when I decided to call you. I thought you, of all the people I knew, could do it and then the Virgin would cry for us all.

Excerpt from the play Virgin Tears by Mary Miller

May 25th

Writing the Dialogue: Your call is important.

These are probably the most hated words in the English language, because we all know our call is not important. Our call is a nuisance. They don't want to take our call. They are not interested in what we think. We are not important … at least not to them. I think that's what makes the statement so irritating. They will get to our call as soon as they can and do what they can when they can. I feel sorry for the innocent person on the other end of the line who finally has to answer the call after we've been waiting 45 minutes or more. This is the drama and stress we endure every day. This is the drama and stress that takes a toll on our health. Next time, when you know you are going to be on hold for a while, decide to create your own diversion, figure out something constructive to do. After all, while your call may not be important to them … your time is important to you.

FRAN: How long do you think we'll have to wait?

ALLISON: I don't know.

FRAN: I hate waiting.

LOUISE: I feel like I've been waiting all my life.

Excerpt from the play <u>Waiting for Oprah</u> by Mary Miller

May 26th

Acting the Part: Disappointment

I think the biggest toll on our health is disappointment. We can overcome just about anything … sickness, loss, pain … but disappointment is something so seemingly small that we can't quite put our finger one it, but it can eat away at our self esteem, our love, our confidence, even our positive outlook on life if we are not careful. We are well equipped to fight the big fight but it's the little fights that we fight every day that sap our strength and drain our energy. Try not to let disappointment ruin your life. You can drown in regret, frustration, and disillusionment. Fight to stay afloat. It might be the most important fight of your life. I know it's the most important fight to win.

ADELE: (puzzled) That car drove right on by.

CHANDLER: (unexpectedly sympathetic) You can't expect every car to stop.

MATTIE: Some people may have given up, gotten disappointed and decided to stay at home.

CANDLER: (speaking from experience) Most people don't have a whole lot of faith when they've been let down a couple of times.

Excerpt from the play Virgin Tears by Mary Miller

May 27th

The Waiting Place

Waiting is a game. Some play it better than others. I know I don't play it well and I'm not sure it's a game you have to play well to win. I do know it's a game we all have to play whether we are waiting for the phone to ring, a day to pass, the news to come, or an answered prayer. We wait and wait and wait and wait. Dr. Seuss in *Oh, The Places You'll Go* described it as a scary place with dark and winding roads. A place you don't want to be. But a place we all visit from time to time.

FRAN: How long do you think we'll have to wait?

ALLISON: I don't know?

FRAN: I hate waiting.

Excerpt from the play <u>Waiting for Oprah</u> by Mary Miller

May 28th

Realism

Realism is just another way to say "no." If someone is realistic chances are they are pessimistic. What is realism anyway? If you are realistic you probably didn't think we could go to the moon in the 1960's. You probably didn't think we could fly an airplane back in the 1900's. You probably didn't think anything could replace the horse back in the 1800's. You never would have dreamed of an Internet that can communicate with the world. Being realistic is being stuck in the times you are living. Fortunately there are people who are not realistic and see the future for what it can be rather than what it isn't. If you find yourself being realistic ... think again about the character you want to play and make a choice to say "Yes, I can" rather than "No, that's not realistic."

MASON: Oh, come on L.E. haven't you ever believed in anything you couldn't explain?

L.E.: (with a sense of loss) I used to believe there were fairies in the mountains - until my Daddy pointed out to me that it was just the reflection of headlights in the mica in the rocks. (pause) Which is exactly what this is going to turn out to be. (abruptly to Merrillee) Are you going to eat any of this, Merrillee, or am I going to have to throw it away to o!

Excerpt from the play <u>Light Burgers</u> by Mary Miller

May 29ᵗʰ

The Golden Rule

In listening to Karen Armstrong discuss The Golden Rule (TED Talk) it struck me because instead of using the positive approach of "Do unto others as you would have them do unto you." She used the negative, and for me even more powerful, approach of "Do not do unto others that which you would not have them do unto you." Technically it means the same thing. But in practice it is easier for me to get my head around what I don't want rather than what I do want. What I do want often drifts into the realm of dreams and wishes. What I don't want is rooted in solid concrete reality. I know what I don't want, and in knowing that, I know what not to do to others to have peace and harmony in the world.

CHILD: But I love you.

WOMAN: That ain't enough. Child ... child, you gots to love me so much that the only color you see is the color of my heart. And I got to love you the same. And we got to take proper care to treat people right, that's the only way we be able to live together ...

Excerpt from the play <u>Take Proper Care</u> by Mary Miller

May 30th

Just say AHHHH,

Or in my world, just say Acting Healthy (A.H. – get it?) … because if you practice acting healthy chances are you will begin to be healthier. It's a fact. What you focus on you will achieve. That's why we shouldn't be surprised when the person who says they are going to fail fails and the person who says they are going to win wins. It's a done deal from the start. We are what we say we are, whether we believe it or not. So, why not say you are healthy, wealthy, and wise. What have you got to lose? Ahhhhhh!

DORIE: Once I had this art teacher named Miss Thumb, who was missing two fingers. She used to say to paint all you needed were your ten good fingers and she'd hold up eight.

Excerpt from the play Ferris Wheel by Mary Miller

May 31st

Batting a 1000?

Batting 1000 is impossible. Nobody bats 1000. That's getting a hit every time you stepped up to the plate. Nobody even bats 500. That's getting a hit almost every other pitch. The best most major league ballplayers hit is 300 and they are lucky to do that. (And those who can are paid millions of dollars!) Hitting 300 is averaging 3 hits for every 10 tries. That's actually missing the ball 7 out of 10 times! So why do we expect a hit every time we put ourselves out? Why do we consider ourselves failures if we fail to bat 1000 or 500 or 300? Give yourself a break. Give yourself a chance. You don't have to be perfect to play in the major leagues! You just have to step up to the plate.

GEORGE: Well, I'm planning on cashing in on this light thing, no matter what anybody says. I got t-shirts, key rings, bumper stickers, novelty items all reading "I Saw The Light" at the Home of the Light Cafe with directions on how to get here printed on the back. I'm even thinking of setting up a UFO Hot Line. Dial-1-900-I.C.A.- U.F.O.2.

Excerpt from the play <u>Light Burgers</u> by Mary Miller

June 1st

New beginnings.

It's summer and it's time to let go of winter and embrace the sun. It's time to get up and go out (to the beach if you can!) As a kid, summer was heaven for me. I loved the hot weather and the long summer days. I loved school being over and having three months off. I loved June, July, and August. But the first day of June was the day I looked forward to the most, because it marked the beginning of the season and anything was possible. Embrace today and go out and do something you used to do as a kid. After all it is the beginning of the season and anything is possible ... again.

The beginning of June marked the beginning of the upfront buying season for EMN. After the major networks announced their new fall schedules and started selling advertising time, EMN followed suit. From June to July EMN would offer up to seventy-five percent of their available commercial advertising time for the coming year to prospective advertising agencies at packaged discount rates. It was the time of year that most major deals were either made or broken. It was the first time McKenzie had more than two or three accounts to work with.

Excerpt from the book A Matter of Grace by Mary Miller

June 2nd

Happy Anniversary!

Today happens to be my parents wedding anniversary! They have been married over sixty years. Congratulations are in order!! Theirs is a truly long running show, which goes to prove that good things can last! Over the years the stage they set for themselves has changed. Their cast of characters have expanded with children and friends ... and in recent years also contracted with loss and death. In their eyes you can see the circle of life reflected time and time again. It has been a gift to be able to watch them and learn from them. Love. Patience. Friendship. Respect. A true partnership. I believe that's the value of a long running show ... what it can teach you as a participant and as an audience member. Happy Anniversary!

ABIGAIL: Fred, I'm sorry about all those things I said. I didn't mean them. It's just when I saw this house it reminded me so much of our old home I didn't think I had the strength to do it all over again. It took thirty-five years to finish that house. I don't have thirty-five years left to build this one.

FRED: You don't have to. We'll just finish it off room by room...

FRED & ABIGAIL: (together) ... as we need them.

Excerpt from the play <u>A Christmas House</u> by Mary Miller

June 3rd

Step Off the Stage

How do you step off the stage you are on? The first thing is to realize you can! I know! I've done it!! It happened in New York City when we were doing the Off Broadway Premier of my play *Light Burgers*. In the middle of the run, I had to take over the role of Merrillee when Lisa Peluso had to do a night shoot for the soap opera *Loving*. It was the weirdest thing, I literally had to enter a diner that I had just imagined, surrounded by people who only existed on paper, and play a character I created in my mind. That was when I realized it was possible!! Yes, you can step off the stage you are on and step onto any stage you want.

MERRILLEE: I used to be in beauty pageant contests all the time as a little bitty girl. Every year Mamma entered me in the Little Miss Sunbeam Contests until I got too tall, broke the height barrier and had to be disqualified. But she took me to every one and used to stay up all night curling my hair. It was a long time before I realized I didn't have naturally curly hair.

Excerpt from the play <u>Light Burgers</u> by Mary Miller

June 4th

Take a mulligan.

A mulligan in golf is known as a do-over. It's another chance to get it right. Taking a mulligan in golf is a practice I think we should adopt in life. It could make a big difference in our lives. We all make mistakes. We all deserve to take a mulligan now and then. We do it all the time in theatre…we just call it rehearsals!

ABIGAIL: You've built the same house. You realize that, don't you?

FRED: It's not exactly the same. It's better!

Excerpt from the play A Christmas House by Mary Miller

June 5th

Continuing Education

You want a better life? Write a better play! The best way I know how to begin is to continue your education. Whether that means getting your GED, or going for a Masters Degree, taking evening classes at a community college, or joining a book club. You should always be looking for ways to grow as a person, and increasing your knowledge and awareness is key to that growth. Look for things that interest you and sign up … who knows you could find new friends, new careers, even a new way to look at your old life.

FRAN: If you vote on whether to continue the book club … I vote YES.

Excerpt from the play <u>Waiting for Oprah</u> by Mary Miller

June 6th

Soul Mate

A lot of stories in theatre and movies revolve around the existence of a soul mate. Now I don't know if I believe in soul mates. In reality it's difficult to get my head around the fact that of the millions of people on Earth we have only a single soul mate. Those who have found theirs will argue the point that they do exist. Those who haven't will argue that they don't. I don't know but I'm willing to hope that a soul mate exists … call me a romantic. I love stories where true love wins in the end. Why not? It makes me feel hopeful and where hope is alive anything can happen.

MERRILLEE: If you ask me Mason is waiting for you to look him in the eye before he can truly be home.

Excerpt from the play Light Burgers by Mary Miller

June 7th

New & Improved

Why is it every time I get use to something they have to update it, upgrade it, change it, and improve it? I'm not at all sure the new and improved is better than the old and proven. I think it's a marketing gimmick and these days I'm more inclined to look for the product that's not marked New & Improved. It's not that I don't want the best; I'm just not convinced that the newest is the best or that we need all this upgrading. Maybe it's just me, or maybe it's just age ... but I'd like a little more time to get use to something before I have to update it, upgrade it, and improve it.

Domino's was running a marketing campaign touting their new and improved pizza that would culminate in December with Santa Claus delivering them throughout the country for those lucky viewers who sent in coupons.

Excerpt from the book A Matter of Grace by Mary Miller

June 8th

Survival of the Fittest

Part of Darwin's Theory of Evolution embraces the idea of the survival of the fittest. The species that is best 'fit' for their environment will be the species that survives. It is also a term used in life ... but it takes on a very cold edge when you apply it to people. Personally, I've found to survive in life you don't always have to lead the charge, sometimes to survive it's best to hunker down, and wait for the storm to pass before making a move. Life can be hard, it can be unfair but if you embrace it and stay engaged it's also possible to survive and maybe even thrive.

BERNICE: I went off again, didn't I?

CLARICE: Just for a second.

BERNICE: I've started to do that recently.

Excerpt from the play <u>Mulberry Lane</u> by Mary Miller

June 9th

Antiques Roadshow PBS

If the Antiques Roadshow isn't theatre then I don't know theatre! It has all the elements of suspense, drama, money, luck, love, and loss. It's a show for everyone because everyone has something in the attic that's old and should be worth something. I love to watch the show. It's fun to compare what the 'contestants' bring to what I actually own. Of course they don't tell you who'll buy the stuff once it's appraised. But we all feel good because what was worthless junk is now priceless antiques. If only we could look at life that way. In a world seemingly obsessed with youth … it's great to have something like the Antiques Roadshow to show us that value does come with age.

MAN: Put it back! It's not like you took a watch or a ring. It's a shirt. They are going to notice. She is lying there without a shirt.

Excerpt from the play Patterson's by Mary Miller

June 10th

Lighten the Load

Sometimes the only way to get ahead in life is to lighten the load you are carrying. Step away from some of the responsibilities you have acquired over the years. Look around … I'm sure there are people who would be happy to assume these responsibilities. Give them a chance to test their wings and see if they can fly. Sometimes we fight giving up control, because we think of it as a loss. But sometimes giving up control can free us to do the things we want to do. If you find you no longer have time to do the things you love, let go of some the things you do, and you'll find the time. Lighten your load. It might be the best for everyone around you, including yourself.

ADELE: I could use your help. I was thinking about going through the house … cleaning it out … getting rid of everything and starting over. I can't do it by myself. It's an old house but it wasn't a bad place to live, was it?

Excerpt from the play <u>Virgin Tears</u> by Mary Miller

June 11th

The Value of a Story.

There is value in telling your life story even if the only person who hears it is you! Telling your life story gives you a distance and a perspective you don't always have when you are in the middle of living it. So, tell your story ... and tell it not only from your point of view but from the vantage point of those in your surrounding cast as well. After all we are not alone in our life stories, even though it often feels that way. And if you can see your life through someone else's eyes, you might find there's more value to your life than you think.

CHANDLER: No. I'm fine. It's OK. It's just strange. Being here. In this house. In this room. (she squints her eyes and looks out) If I close my eyes and tilt my head, just so, I can still see my bulletin board with a white corsage pinned to it, my blue relay ribbons, campaign buttons, high school medals, and that old orange haired troll doll I hung for luck. "Good luck, Chandler." (she opens her eyes and looks at Mattie) I remember my 13th birthday; Momma gave me a LadyBug light-blue-pleated-button-down-shirt-waist dress. (pleased) I was a girl ready to be a woman. A child fantasizing about the future.

Excerpt from the play <u>Virgin Tears</u> by Mary Miller

June 12th

Enthusiasm

You can't manufacture it but you can fake it. If you fake it long enough you'll believe it. At least that's what the experts say. But my theory is this … if you fake it long enough you will find a solution that will lead to real enthusiasm. See the difference? There's a step in between faking it and making it and it's called finding it. By faking it you will find, stumble, trip, fall over the answers you need. It may not be a pretty process but in the end you'll get that 'genius' idea that will enable you to survive whatever crisis, calamity, or disaster may befall you. Enthusiasm fake it until you find it!

DORIE: My Mother always said it was our social obligation to be entertaining.

Excerpt from the play <u>Ferris Wheel</u> by Mary Miller

June 13th

Cutting the dialogue.

Sometimes you have to cut your favorite part to make the whole better. The easiest way to see this is in a script. From a distance anybody can tell when the dialogue in a play or movie goes off track. It's not so easy when you are in the thick of playing the part and you treasure every word. The same is true in life. Sometimes the less said the better. Hold your thoughts before putting everything into words. Reflection can be the better part of valor. My momma used to say, think before you speak. It was true then and it's true now.

JANICE: There wasn't one speck of traffic. Do you think the media knows she's coming?

LOUISE: Janice, you didn't tell the local news did you? I hope you didn't tell! We're not supposed to tell anyone!

Excerpt from the play Waiting for Oprah by Mary Miller

June 14th

Bully This!

Bullies exist is all shapes and sizes. They span all age ranges. You know a true bully by the way they'll hit you when you are down. Do you ignore them? Stand to them? Fight them? Run from them? It's hard to say because it's easier to be mean these days than it's ever been before. My thought, try and find a way around the bullies in your life. Go over them, under them, around them, and even through them if you have too. Build on your strengths … it will give you a leg to stand on.

L.E.: Merrillee, has he hit you?

MERRILLEE: He doesn't mean to. It's my fault. I aggravate him. The way I look. The way I breathe. The sound of my voice. I suppose we never should have gotten married. Isn't it funny what you will do to make other people happy.

Excerpt from the play Light Burgers by Mary Miller

June 15th

Make Up!

In Vaudeville shows you'll often hear a cry for MAKE UP and somebody gets hit in the face with an oversized powder puff! It's a joke. It gets the audience laughing and brings the show back to life. It's interesting when you think about it. When things go wrong on stage they call for make up ... as if by reapplying make up they get to start over again. Maybe it's true. Make up is a wonderful thing. We girls have known that for years. But I don't know if people think of it in healing terms. If you're feeling down ... redo your make up. Anybody at a department store can help you. Let them pamper you and study you. Let them give you a new face. See yourself though someone else's eyes. It may give you a fresh look at the make up of your life.

MERRILLEE: How do I look? No shine on my nose...no lipstick on my teeth...

Excerpt from the play Light Burgers by Mary Miller

June 16th

Persistence

When things don't work … try, try, try again. I have been taught this since birth (at least as far back as I can remember!) But, these days, I often forget how important it is to keep trying. Sometimes I think we feel so overwhelmed that we give up before we even get started. It seems the smallest obstacle can derail us. I can't tell you why … but I can tell you this: persistence works. It worked then and it will work now. Don't give up. Try one more time and then try again.

DOWNSTAIRS: Why don't you just stop?

UPSTAIRS: I want my name in that book!

Excerpt from the play <u>At 3:00 O'clock in the Morning</u> by Mary Miller

June 17th

Hearing Music

When people talk about marching to the sound of a different drum … this is what they mean. They hear a different internal music that defines the life they live. There is music all around us, inside and out. We talk in rhythms whether it's Southern, Northern, Midwestern, you name it. Yes, the lines differentiating the dialects are blurring and in some cases they've disappeared all together. But there is music in our souls. Listen carefully. You'll know it when you hear it … it's a beautiful sound.

CLARICE: Hey, what about a musical?

Excerpt from the play <u>Mulberry Lane</u> by Mary Miller

June 18th

The Need to Lose

In life there are winners and losers. As much fun as it is to win, it can be important to lose. I've found that most real winners have lost something at some point in their life. I think losing might be a perquisite to winning. In losing you discover what's important in your life and the lengths you'll go to fight for it. Losing can define who you are … it highlights your strengths and your weaknesses. My mother used to say "losing builds character." It wasn't a very comforting thought then but I understand it better now. Losing often gives you the character to win.

JOHN: But you filled out nicely.

DORIE: (embarrassed) Thank you.

JOHN: (distracted) A regular beauty pageant contestant.

DORIE: I was once. But I didn't win.

JOHN: The prettiest girl doesn't always win.

Excerpt from the play Ferris Wheel by Mary Miller

June 19th

The Art of Pretending

As an actress there are many schools of thought on how to act, but for me the best way was through the art of pretending. I didn't have to have experienced everything my character had in order to portray her. I just pretended. You don't have to worry about how well you act to act healthy. You just have to pretend for a moment and let that moment last as long as it can. You'll find pretending gets easier the more you do it. If you pretend you feel well, chances are you will begin to feel better.

MATTIE: Don't you think we are a little too old to set sail in the Merry MAC?

CHANDLER: You're never too old to set sail in an imaginary boat!

Excerpt from the play <u>Virgin Tears</u> by Mary Miller

June 20th

Love

Love is a word that gets bantered about a lot. It's written on t-shirts, in greeting cards, on billboards, and tattooed on skin. But what does the word really mean? Webster defines it as an intense affection for another person. But to me, love is compassion ... empathy ... the ability to put yourself in the shoes of someone else and see the world through their eyes.

CHILD: I want to go with you.

WOMAN: You can't child. It don't matter how hard you try. There are some things in this world you just can't change.

CHILD: But I love you.

Excerpt from the play <u>Take Proper Care</u> by Mary Miller

June 21st

Give it up!

Let go of the things you no longer need or use. Throw them away. Or at least give them away. You can't take them with you. Of course we know this in theory but I swear there are people out there who believe there's a luggage rack on a hearse. There isn't! We come into this world with nothing and we leave it with nothing. So ask yourself, do you own your possessions or do they own you? If it's the later, take control over your world and give them up!!

BERNICE: Clarice, you stay away from my closet!

CLARICE: Bernice, it's junk and I'm throwing it away!

Excerpt from the play <u>Mulberry Lane</u> by Mary Miller

June 22nd

What matters most?

Sometimes what matters most is the most difficult thing in life to figure out. Some days it can change by the hour; you start the morning with one thought and end the day with another. What mattered last year may no longer be an issue today. It's funny when you step back and look at the bigger picture. Most of us will agree that people matter more ... but then we focus on things. Take a second look at what matters most in your life and take time to pay attention to them

FRAN: It doesn't matter. I don't care where he was—it's where he is that matters now.

Excerpt from the play <u>Waiting for Oprah</u> by Mary Miller

June 23rd

Walk in my shoes.

There's an old Biblical passage that talks about walking a mile in someone else's shoes before you can judge them. I think we forget to do this in our busy hurry up world. We don't want to walk anywhere ... much less is someone else's shoes! But if you can, for a moment, the one thing I'll tell you is it will give you a whole different perspective on the life you are living ... and the shoes you are wearing!

JANICE: Well, I can't wait much longer ... not in these shoes.

(Janice kicks off her high heels ... they slide across the floor.)

Excerpt from the play <u>Waiting for Oprah</u> by Mary Miller

June 24th

Words matter.

What you say matters. Words make a difference. They make a difference to your family, your friends, your co-workers, and you! What you say, and how you say it, not only impacts your health and wellbeing, it impacts the health and wellbeing of everyone around you. Be careful what you say ... words matter.

CHANDLER: You could have told me.

ROBERT: Not at first. I couldn't tell anyone. Then after a while it didn't seem to matter.

CHANDLER: It matters.

Excerpt from the play Virgin Tears by Mary Miller

June 25th

The End

These are the two most powerful words in the English language. Because they mark the end of what is often a very long journey. Whether it is physical or spiritual, real or imagined. The End is the final moment. The moment when the hero either succeeds or fails. The moment when you either win or lose. But no matter which, *The End*, also marks the point of a new beginning.

BERNICE: Will you be here when I get back?

CLARICE: You don't need me anymore, you old goat, now go on get the hell out of here.

Excerpt from the play <u>Mulberry Lane</u> by Mary Miller

June 26th

Delete

Sometimes you just have to hit the delete button to get rid of the junk in your life. Personally I've got years worth of e-mails from people I don't even know anymore that are cluttering up my in box. I think it may have something to do with hitting "delete" and then being asked if I'm sure I want to permanently delete it from my life. I'm not sure I want to permanently delete anything but it's time to make room for something new. Hit delete and move on!

CHANDLER: I have to quit my job. Do something else. Get out of there while people still think I'm worth working with, at this rate it's hard to tell who's crazier. Me or my boss.

Excerpt from the play <u>Virgin Tears</u> by Mary Miller

June 27th

The right time?

So often we put our life on hold waiting for the right time, the right place, the right person. We are so busy waiting we don't get a chance to experience life. The problem with waiting for the right time, is that by the time you know it, it's past. Waiting for the right place, by the time you find it, it's gone. Waiting for the right person, they're taken. I'm not advocating settling for less; I'm just saying give up the search for perfect ... the right time is now.

CHANDLER: I always expected to marry you, Bobby. Somewhere in the back of my mind, it's always been a possibility ... a probability. But I was such a moving target ...

ROBERT: (interrupting her) Chandler don't.

CHANDLER: (embarrassed) Look at me. I come back into town and the first thing I do is propose to my old high school boyfriend. Living in the big city you learn to spot what you want and take it – or at least ask for it.

Excerpt from the play <u>Virgin Tears</u> by Mary Miller

June 28th

Writing the Dialogue: "Thank you"

"Thank you" - are two words that can move mountains. They can soften hearts. Change minds. Motivate a team. Alter the direction of your life! The problem is we don't say them enough. You have to practice saying the words you want, in order to be able to say them when they matter most. "Thank you" is one of the most underrated expressions because we often think it goes without saying ... but that's not true ... it needs to be said. Whether someone gives you a hand, helps you at work, or literally saves your life. "Thank you" goes a long way in bridging the gap between what you have and what you want.

MASON: I think George has done a good job.

GEORGE: Why, thank you, Mason.

MASON: You're welcome.

Excerpt from the play <u>Light Burgers</u> by Mary Miller

June 29th

Writing the Dialogue: "I'm sorry"

They say "I'm sorry" are the two hardest words in the English language to say ... and some people can go a lifetime without ever saying them. I don't know why ... except I believe some people think saying "I'm sorry" is a sign of weakness. It's not. If anything it's a sign of strength. To be sorry, truly sorry for something you did, and be able to say that to the person you've wronged, goes a long way in making the two of you better, healthier, and happier. It may be naive but I honestly believe if more people were able to say "I'm sorry" the world would be a better place to live.

CHANDLER: Mattie, I'm sorry.

MATTIE: For what?

CHANDLER: Everything.

Excerpt from the play Virgin Tears by Mary Miller

June 30th

Writing the Dialogue: "I love you"

These may be the most overused words in the English language unless they are being spoken to you! "I love you" can cover a multitude of sins. It's the balm when we are hurt. It's the reason we marry. It gives us the strength to start over. "I love you" are the three words we all long to hear. Practice saying them to yourself in the mirror. You'll not only learn how to say them out loud .. you might find that you actually begin to fall in love with yourself.

ABIGAIL: I love you.

FRED: I know. You want to see her?

ABIGAIL: I might faint again.

FRED: I'll catch you.

Excerpt from the play <u>A Christmas House</u> by Mary Miller

July 1ˢᵗ

Quitting

Do you know the reason 99% of people fail? They quit too soon. If you research the big success stories throughout history you'll find there were always several people working on the same idea at the same time. The reason some people succeeded while others failed was the fact that those who failed quit. It is said that Thomas Edison failed 1000 times before he finally created a light bulb that worked. If you believe in what you are doing keep doing it. Quitters never win and winners never quit. And guess what, once you've succeeded, everyone will think you are a genius … too!

GEORGE: *A man has to do what a man has to do.*

Excerpt from the play <u>Light Burgers</u> by Mary Miller

July 2nd

Motivation

There are three things that can motivate anyone into action. They are fame, fortune, and love. Most actors are seeking all three if they are honest with themselves! But the truth is we all need fame, fortune, and love to a certain degree. We need them to survive. Think of fame as encouragement and recognition. Fortune as a wage or a salary. Love as love for a job as well as one another. These are key motivating forces because they are three key ingredients of life!

CLARICE: (proudly) I had my moments on stage.

BERNICE: You can't live off moments.

CLARICE: You can't live without 'em.

Excerpt from the play <u>Mulberry Lane</u> by Mary Miller

July 3rd

Air conditioning!

This time of year is so hot it can steam the life right out of you ... if you're not careful. Did you know the invention that made summer bearable and productive was air conditioning? It's true. Can you imagine trying to get through the summer without it? Can you imagine trying to get through the day without it? Can you imagine putting on a show even at night without it? In the summer we slow down because it's hot. Air conditioning made it possible to function. Try air conditioning your mind ... and cool down some of those hot angry thoughts that can keep you from functioning spring, summer, winter, and fall!

PEARL: (wiping her brow) Whew, it's hot for 9:30 at night. (pause) What do you guess the temperature is? 80 - 90 degrees?

RUTH: Could be. Doesn't feel one bit cooler than it did this afternoon. The air conditioner went out at work. I thought I'd die. Everybody sitting in a building with no air and the windows sealed shut.

Excerpt from the play I Witness by Mary Miller

July 4th

Freedom

Freedom it means different things to different people. To some, freedom is so real they can touch it. Freedom from debt. Freedom from hunger. Freedom from pain. To others freedom is more intangible ... an idea or a belief. Freedom to pursue a dream. Freedom to be who you want to be. Whatever freedom means to you, the 4th of July is the time when everyone in the United States celebrates it together. Freedom. Something to celebrate!

CHILD: What time is it now?

WOMAN: It must be going on five ... five thirty.

CHILD: A half hour of freedom left.

Excerpt from the play Take Proper Care by Mary Miller

July 5th

Times a wasting…

Do you realize we are now exactly six months into the New Year? Did you know that by the 5th of January almost everyone who made a New Year's Resolution broke it? It's a fact most New Year's resolution don't last more than a week. So why do I bring this up now? Because at this half way point in the year why not renew your New Year's Resolution? You still have six months left to make a difference in your life. If it was a good idea then it's probably still a good idea now? Go ahead and do it today … times a wasting!

MATTIE: Will you stop teasing her?

CHANDLER: Who's teasing?!

(Chandler looks at Mattie and smiles.)

MATTIE: Come on, we've got chairs to get and times a wasting.

Excerpt from the play <u>Virgin Tears</u> by Mary Miller

July 6th

Daylight Savings Time

I love this time of year because it stays light until after 9:00 p.m. and I feel like I have two days in one. You see the first eight hours of my day I work. But the next eight hours I can play outside in the sunlight. I can do whatever I like. Play golf or tennis. Go to the beach and read. See a concert in the park. People can spend quality time with their families because of Daylight Savings Time. I know some purest complain that we are messing with the laws of nature. But time is really a manufactured way of measuring the day and as for me I love the extra time I get in my day during the summer months.

MERRILLEE: They are waiting for the light.

GEORGE: It's not even dark. You'd think they'd come in by now, order something, eat and avoid the evening rush!

Excerpt from the play Light Burgers by Mary Miller

July 7th

Sands of Time

If you are fortunate enough to have the opportunity to take a vacation, I suggest going to the beach … any beach and take a long walk beside the ocean. Feel the sand between your toes and look out to sea … it's closest thing we have to time travel today. Think about it. The view you have now of the ocean is the same as it was years and years ago. The sand beneath your feet is the same sand people walked on long before you were born. If you want to know what it was like a hundred years ago take a walk by the ocean and the sands of time disappear.

JACKSON: Sometimes, I hold my hand out into the night and it disappears in the darkness.

Excerpt from the play I Witness by Mary Miller

July 8th

Taken for granted.

We often take things for granted until we are confronted with the loss of those things we love … whether they be people, possessions, health, or wealth … a loss puts everything in perspective. Wouldn't it be great if we could appreciate what we have while we have it. Loss is a favorite subject for drama. It heightens the stakes and gives value to what remains. Today try to give thanks for what you have without taking anything for granted.

CLAIRE: Ordinarily I don't think about it. I took them for granted. That they'd always be there. It was just something I expected to see every morning when I woke up. Like an arm or a leg. Nothing particularly romantic or sexy but a part of me nonetheless.

Excerpt from the play <u>NEXT</u> by Mary Miller

July 9th

Plan ahead…?

Good advice, if you're smart enough to take it. But let's face it most of us aren't. Try as we will, we often go off half cocked with no idea where we'll end up. Of course, everyone will tell you that's not the way to live your life. But sometimes what you don't plan for can be the best thing you get. Sometimes we plan the life out of things. Sometimes it might be best to sit back and let circumstances take you where they will. I know as a writer the more I try to control what I'm writing the harder it is to write. Give up a little control and you may get more than you ever could if you planned everything ahead.

LOUISE: Oh, Allison! You've redone everything!?! You didn't do this just for today?

ALLISON: Not everything. When was the last time you were here?

LOUISE: I guess it's been a while. You've been busy!

ALLISON: I've had time.

LOUISE: Allison, I could have all the time in the world. I couldn't do this.

Excerpt from the play <u>Waiting for Oprah</u> by Mary Miller

July 10th

Clear polish…

When doing your nails they end each treatment with a coat of clear polish. This helps smooth out the rough spots and gives your fingers a shine that sparkles. Now I'm not an advocate for polishing over everything. But every now and then I think a clear coat of polish could go a long way in smoothing a multitude of sins … particularly in what we say and do to one another.

WOMAN: We got to take proper care to treat people right, that's the only way we be able to live together … you and me and Mary Lou O'Callahan …

Excerpt from the play <u>Take Proper Care</u> by Mary Miller

July 11th

Celebrate Good Times

"Celebrate … good times!" is a line in a song that keeps running through my mind. It's a special song they usually sing for special events. But as it continues to play in my head, I'm thinking why not sing it in the morning when you first wake up? "Celebrate" … you're alive. "Good times" … are still ahead. "Celebrate Good Times!" It may be the perfect alarm clock!!

Monday morning came early. It always did. It was funny how after the weekend and two days of sleeping in McKenzie's internal clock switched off. By Wednesday she'd wake up on her own before the blaring of the alarm clock but not on Mondays.

Excerpt from the book <u>A Matter of Grace</u> by Mary Miller

July 12th

Infinite Intelligence

Whether you call it God or not … I do believe there is such a thing as infinite intelligence. I believe it every time I step on a stage. Whether I am portraying someone who lived in real life or totally fictional I feel the power of infinite intelligence informing my every move. Also as a writer when I'm stuck I often look to the heavens for inspiration. It's a request to infinite intelligence to help me find an answer. To me it's comforting to believe in the power of infinite intelligence particularly in these times when answers seem to be so few and far between.

CHANDLER: Adele! If that is God we're all doomed. We all might as well take a rope and hang in Daddy's closet cause we haven't got a prayer. We have to believe there's something bigger on this earth than a bathtub Virgin crying real tears? We have to have faith that our tears count too.

Excerpt from the play <u>Virgin Tears</u> by Mary Miller

July 13th

When you are ready.

Psychologists have said, "when someone is truly ready for something that *something* usually appears." I'm not sure if this is always true but it does make sense. In a way it's like opening a door that was previously closed. When you are ready you open doors to new people, places, and things.

UPSTAIRS: They welcome direct contributions from new record breakers. It's in the book. Look it up. HUMAN ACHIEVEMENTS "Endurance and Endeavors."

Excerpt from the play <u>At Three O'clock In The Morning</u> by Mary Miller

July 14th

Opportunity knocks?

It has been my experience that opportunity doesn't always knock. Would that it did!! Opportunity can be elusive and difficult to pin down. It can be hard to recognize and can come in the form of failure! If opportunity came knocking who among us wouldn't open the door and welcome it into our lives. No we have to seek out opportunities like a needle in a haystack ... with our eyes wide open and a willingness to look for it.

RUTH: Pearl, this could be Jackson's opportunity to get us out of here.

JACKSON: All of us. Every last one of us!!

Excerpt from the play I Witness by Mary Miller

July 15th

Act on it.

When you get an idea the best suggestion I can give you is to act on it. Who knows where ideas come from? Usually they just pop out of nowhere and usually those ideas are the best ideas because they come from somewhere outside ourselves. If you listen to people who have written great literature or composed beautiful music … they'll often say the idea came to them in a flash or a dream. But be aware just because an idea came to you in an instant it may take you lifetime to fulfill it. Do yourself a favor when you get an idea act on it now … it may be the most exciting adventure of your life.

BABS: WAIT! WAIT!! Don't go! I've got an idea. I have an IDEA!!

Excerpt from the play <u>A Christmas House</u> by Mary Miller

July 16th

Getting to yes.

Sometimes the only way to get to *yes* is by never taking *no* for an answer. Success comes through sheer persistence of will. It's funny but before anything is possible it always seems impossible. You can ask anyone … but don't. You don't need everyone's opinion to succeed. In fact most people's opinions are usually negative, particularly when it comes to doing something new and different with your life. So in my opinion … the best way to get to yes is to surround yourself with people who are positive and never take no for an answer.

JANICE: WHERE IS SHE!?

LOUISE: She is coming! Mark my words. When Oprah sets her mind to do something, she does it. We all could take a page out of Oprah's book.

Excerpt from the play Waiting for Oprah by Mary Miller

July 17th

Creating suspense.

The best way to create suspense for an audience is by posing a question and then making them wait for an answer. Create a problem and work towards the solution. The key is to never let your audience get ahead of you. Once they know the answer. Once they've solved the problem ... the drama is over. Move fast and ask the next question before your audience heads for the door.

JOHN: Excuse me. Excuse me? I hope I'm not ... crowding you?

Excerpt from the play Ferris Wheel by Mary Miller

July 18th

Polish your shoes.

My mother always told me to wear clean underwear incase I was ever in an accident. My advice to you is to always polish your shoes whenever you go on an audition or interview. People will judge you by the shoes you wear. They will! Whether you believe it or not it's all part of the costume. Remember they'll be studying you from head to toe. Make sure your shoes are cleaned and polished it's the last step in making a good first impression.

LOUISE: Hello feet. Wow, I wonder when was the last time I noticed my feet?

Excerpt from the play Waiting for Oprah by Mary Miller

July 19th

So hot!

Some days it's just too hot to move. Some days it's best to stay inside, drink a tall glass of sweet tea and read a good book. That is if you don't have to go to work! Some days are too hot to do anything but sit … and that's a good thing. Some days we should stop what we are doing and take time to relax. It will be cold soon enough.

RUTH: You want that fan blowing directly on you or you mind if it oscillates 'round the room a bit?

Excerpt from the play <u>I Witness</u> by Mary Miller

July 20th

Powerful Thoughts

Do you know that you have the power to control your thoughts? It's the greatest power you own. But it's a power few people use because they don't know how to develop it. Thinking is a muscle … use it or lose it! Really!! The more you think, the more you are capable of thinking. The more you are capable of thinking, the more you can control your thoughts. This is important to know because your body responds to the thoughts you are thinking regardless of whether your thoughts are positive or negative. If you ask me, it's much more powerful, helpful, and beneficial to your over all wellbeing to think positive … the trick is learning to control what you think.

JANICE: I say The Prayer of Jabez every morning. Then wait to see what I get.

LOUISE: That's not the point of the prayer?

JANICE: So far it's working. So don't say another word. You might jinx it.

Excerpt from the play <u>Waiting for Oprah</u> by Mary Miller

July 21st

Desire

Desire is the key to getting what you want. Notice I didn't say *wish* ... I said *want*. You can wish all day long but until you want something bad enough with a burning desire to get it ... your want will remain a wish forever and ever.

The past year had been hard because she had spent a good deal of it alone. A little over a year ago, Fred, her husband of thirty-five years, began building a beach house on an island off the southern tip of the coast of Georgia with money he had inherited from his ninety-five year old mother. When he first told Abigail about his plans, she was reluctant to agree. He was a strong man and had been a fine architect, but he was sixty-eight years old at the time, entirely too old to start building again she thought. And even though it had been his dream for as long as she could remember, it never occurred to her that when he bought the land he would build the house.

Excerpt from the book <u>A Christmas House</u> by Mary Miller

July 22nd

Costumes

I have to admit I went through a down period in my life where I didn't care what I wore or how it looked. In this day and age it's easy to get away with it. Everyone wants to be comfortable but comfortable isn't synonymous with success. I don't mean you have to go out and buy a whole new wardrobe but a few new pieces would go a long way in making a difference. Remember if costumes didn't matter we wouldn't need a wardrobe department. The actors could wear what they wanted but it wouldn't be always right for the role. Remember when you go out you are playing a part ... why not dress for success.

ALLISON: Does anyone know if they are actually going to film this?

JANICE: They have to! Otherwise, what's the point! I bought a whole new outfit.

Excerpt from the play Waiting for Oprah by Mary Miller

July 23rd

Scenery

If there is anything you want in this life ... paint a picture of it for yourself. I'm not just talking about literally putting paint on a canvas I'm talking about painting a picture with words. Words that are descriptive. Words that are colorful. Words that will bring your pictures to life. Paint a picture of the life you want with words. The more you can picture the scenery in your mind the closer you will be to achieving it in your life

JACKSON: No sir....we gonna move ... far away from here. To a big house ... in the countryside...

(He kisses her neck.)

RUTH: Where trees don't grow out of little cement holes ... bums don't beg...

(Ruth throws her head back in pleasure.)

JACKSON: (CONT) Doors aren't locked ... (he opens her shirt again) ... windows aren't broken...

Excerpt from the play I Witness by Mary Miller

July 24th

A True Mirror

The question here is how do you see yourself? Seriously, when you look in a mirror what do you see? Are you tall, short, thin, fat? If you were a casting director how would you cast yourself? I hate to say it but most people judge people by their appearance. We rarely have time to get to know someone for who they are rather than what they look like. To change the part you're playing ... why not change the way you look? It's easier than you think. First: take a good hard look in the mirror. Second: concentrate on those features you like. Third: decide what you can change and what you can't and then set about making those changes a reality.

LOUISE: I thought about putting out an APB. But how do you put out an All Points Bulletin to find yourself? Call the police and they ask...How long has the person been missing?...I say...Fifteen years! It surprises me I have any reflection at all. When I happen to catch a glimpse of myself in the chrome on the toaster it scares me!

Excerpt from the play <u>Waiting for Oprah</u> by Mary Miller

July 25th

Dream Big Dreams

As a kid I dreamed of being on Broadway, seeing my name up in lights, and living in New York. It was a big dream ... an impossible dream if you asked my friends and family. But what's the point of dreaming if your dreams are too small? If you can get what on your own, there's no need in dreaming at all. So, if you are going to dream, have the courage to dream big. Then, even if you don't get everything you dreamed of ... you'll probably get more than you expected.

ANN: When I was young I used to dream of being famous. I grew up practicing signing my autograph. Ann McKenzie. Famous. Successful. Rich.

Excerpt from the play (A Matter of) Grace by Mary Miller

July 26th

Growing Young

How do you grow young? You laugh. You never feel old when you're laughing. You never look old when you're laughing. Young people will gravitate to you when you laugh, especially when you are old, because they'll want to know the secret to your success!

ANNE: (laughing to Claire) Do you remember those exercises you could do to increase your bra size?

(Anne and Clair both press their hands together in front of their chest as they sing.)

ANNE & CLAIR: "We must. We must. We must increase our bust!"

(They burst out laughing!)

Excerpt from the play <u>NEXT</u> by Mary Miller

July 27th

Step away from the ledge!

When you feel totally overwhelmed try to step back away from the problem. Try to give yourself a moment of peace. A moment to think. A moment to walk away. Because tomorrow is another day and you don't know what tomorrow will bring. Give yourself a second chance ... step away from the ledge.

CHANDLER: Do you think she really tried to kill herself?

MATTIE: I don't know. But what ever happens, don't mention it.

CHANDLER: Don't mention what? The rope. The suicide. The Virgin.

MATTIE: Any of it.

Excerpt from the play <u>Virgin Tears</u> by Mary Miller

July 28th

Setting boundaries.

There are boundaries on the stage just as there should be boundaries in life. On stage we call the boundary between the audience and the actors the fourth wall ... because it can't be seen but should rarely be broken. It's important to set boundaries for yourself in life. Boundaries to protect you from people who would do you harm whether they be inside your family or outside! You can't always build physical walls to protect yourself but you don't have to ... remember the fourth wall in the theatre and let that be your guide.

MASON: In New York it's amazing how close you can stand to someone and how far away you can be.

(L.E. walks away from him and crosses downstage to Merrillee's booth.)

L.E.: I guess if you're not going to know someone ... it's better not knowing them clear across the room.

Excerpt from the play <u>Light Burgers</u> by Mary Miller

July 29th

Look sexy.

The thing about movie stars is they always look sexy on screen and on stage. Of course they have make up artist and wardrobe people hanging on their every move. But you too can look sexy because sexy is a feeling anyone can master. It's a state of mind … not a state of being. To be sexy all you have to be is confident (in everything you say and do!) Be confident enough to look others in the eye. Be confident enough to hold their gaze. Be confident enough to speak softly, lower your voice, and smile. Confidence is sexy. With a little practice anyone can look sexy!

CHANDLER: *The first time I wore this outfit I thought I was so hot. Now it's almost embarrassing to be seen in public in it.*

ROBERT: *I remember it.*

(Chandler smiles and twirls in front of him. It's sexy, despite the style and he is taken with it … and she knows it.)

Excerpt from the play <u>Virgin Tears</u> by Mary Miller

July 30th

Sweet time…

"Take your sweet time" is an expression we say all the time down here in the South. Because down here in the South we know the value of taking time for ourselves. Scientists say the body need 8 hours of sleep a night. I feel lucky if I can get as much as 6 to 7 hours a night! But during the day when I can, I take my sweet time, whenever I can. It's like taking a nap … it refreshes my soul and gives me the energy I need to get through the day.

ALLISON: No, Oprah is not here.

FRAN: Good.

LOUISE: Neither is Mia.

JANICE: She's always late.

ALLISON: It's not like she lives down the street anymore.

Excerpt from the play <u>Waiting for Oprah</u> by Mary Miller

July 31st

Vacation time…

If you haven't all ready I suggest taking a vacation. It's almost the end of the summer and if you haven't gotten out away from the office you're going to need more than a little time later to recover. We often like to think of ourselves as being able to handle anything. But that's not true. We all have breaking points and it's best to take a break before we break. It's the summer after all … go take a vacation!! Even the theatre goes dark, every now and then, to get ready for the next show.

MASON: I think you should go. You could use a vacation.

L.E.: Mason, what?! Did you come back to Dillard just to tell us all how we should be living our lives?

MERRILLEE: A Vacation. Lenora Elaine, you definitely need a vacation.

Excerpt from the play Light Burgers by Mary Miller

August 1st

Storm clouds.

We all can tell when a storm is brewing and I'm not talking about just the weather. You can see the storm clouds rise in people's eyes when they have been hurt. You can hear the thunder roll when a friend's been wronged. You can feel the devastation when a heart's been broken. We learn how to prepare for the storms outside. We buy insurance to replace what's lost. But it's the storm inside that takes us by surprise and no insurance can repair the damage done there. So beware the storm clouds when you see them coming ... seek higher ground and take cover so you can live to fight another day.

ADELE: I hated you for leaving, Chandler! I wondered how you escaped?

(Chandler stops and turns back to Adele.)

CHANDLER: I didn't escape, Adele. I just ran the other way.

Excerpt from the play <u>Virgin Tears</u> by Mary Miller

August 2nd

The sound track of our lives!

Here Comes the Sun was one of my favorite Beatles songs. I loved the music. I loved the words. I loved the memory of driving to the beach listening to it play over and over on a cassette recorder. The beauty of music is what it enables us to feel. What it enables us to remember. Be cognizant of the music in your life's play. It is the sound track of your life, and if you choose well, it can part the clouds and let the sunshine in.

CHANDLER: Do you ever dance anymore, Mattie? Just put on a record and dance? (Chandler stands and starts to hum) Come on.

MATTIE: I can't dance.

CHANDLER: Come on. Like we did as kids on Daddy's feet. Come stand on mine and we'll dance around the house.

Excerpt from the play <u>Virgin Tears</u> by Mary Miller

August 3rd

Time

Today is the tomorrow you worried about yesterday. Understand? The future happens. Days pass. Weeks become months. Months become years. There is no stopping the passing of time. Of course some days seem longer than others, some years go by faster than you can imagine. They say time heals all wounds. That may be true. Time passes no matter what you do, but time only heals if you let it.

PEARL: *What time is it getting to be?*

RUTH: *(looking at her watch) 9:30.*

PEARL: *I thought you said Jackson was coming home for dinner.*

RUTH: *I thought he was.*

PEARL: *What you thought and what's reality, look to be two different things.*

Excerpt from the play <u>I Witness</u> by Mary Miller

August 4th

Bad Hair Day

I used to worry about bad hair days until I met people with cancer. They would give their eye-teeth for one of my bad days. It's funny how we take things for granted ... until we lose them. Losing your hair due to chemo and cancer is one of the most mentally devastating thing about the disease. But take solace in the fact that it will grow back ... and surprisingly to some ... it grows back better.

ALISON: I watched Oprah everyday during the chemo and radiation. I had prayed so hard before for things that never came, I was afraid to pray then to live for fear of dying. So I prayed to Oprah when I couldn't pray to God.

Excerpt from the play <u>Waiting for Oprah</u> by Mary Miller

August 5th

Be the change!

Gandhi once said: "Be the change you want to see in the world." But change is hard. Most people don't want to change. We get comfortable the way we are. We feel lost when things change around us. Old. Irrelevant. Out of place. That's the frightening thing about old age. Like an old tree we become brittle and break. But it's not inevitable. You can change. You just have to make up your mind to play a different part. Change isn't easy, but it's not always bad.

CHANDLER: He hasn't changed.

MATTIE: Yes he has.

ADELE: He used to be a lot more tolerant then he is now!

Excerpt from the play <u>Virgin Tears</u> by Mary Miller

August 6th

Success

Sometimes success is not what we imagine it to be. Sometimes it's better.

ABIGAIL: It's going to be a good house, isn't it, Fred?

FRED: I think so.

Excerpt from the play <u>A Christmas House</u> by Mary Miller

August 7th

Live in the moment.

That's what acting really is, living in the moment, even when you've memorized the lines, rehearsed the play, and played the part for years. That's what it looks like to an audience ... as if you're hearing the information for the first time. Try living in the moment ... you might discover something new.

MATTIE: That must have been a revealing moment.

Excerpt from the play Virgin Tears by Mary Miller

August 8th

Black Box Stage

In theatre there is a type of stage called a Black Box. The walls are black, the floor is black, and the ceiling is black. It's designed that way so any production can come into the space and make it their own. The thing I find fascinating about a black box stage is no matter how elaborate or simple a show may be, at the end of the run, the stage is always repainted black to make it ready for the next production. I like to think of life like a black box stage ... with every ending there is a new beginning. We just paint the stage black and start over again.

ABIGAIL: You know. I did some thinking about this house. All it really needs is some sheetrock and plaster. I can paint ... remember?

FRED: You're a damn fine painter, Abby.

Excerpt from the play <u>A Christmas House</u> by Mary Miller

August 9th

Laughter is the best ... medicine.

I recently read *Anatomy of an Illness* by Norman Cousins. In it he describes how when he was diagnosed with a serious illness he literally locked himself in a room, watched comedies and laughed out loud. It was his cure and his salvation. We forget how powerful a good laugh can be. It's good for the heart. It cleanses the soul. It's great exercise. It doesn't even have to be real to be effective ... so repeat after me: HA HA HE HE HOOOO! Feel better?

JANICE: I started dating again. Don't laugh. He's sort of blue-collar. Works with his hands. I hired him to finish off the back porch.

Excerpt from the play <u>Waiting for Oprah</u> by Mary Miller

August 10th

Computer Hell

I have to keep reminding myself I can't get angry at a computer, it will only make matters worse. Sometimes I believe a computer can sense when I'm at my wits end. It can tell by the pounding on the keys, the gnashing of teeth, and the pulling of hair. (Nowhere else except on stage am I more dramatic!) The thing I have to remember when caught in a struggle for survival with my computer is to take my glasses off, step away, breathe, and turn the damn thing off! Nine times out of ten, that's the solution.

McKenzie slammed the phone down so hard on the receiver; it shattered the computer readout that gave the date, time, and name of the caller.

Excerpt from the book <u>A Matter of Grace</u> by Mary Miller

August 11th

A new beginning.

Not all new beginnings start off with a bang. Not all new beginnings are as monumental as the birth of a child, or a wedding, or getting a new job. Some new beginnings are quiet transitions that enable you to move forward when you didn't think it was possible. Some new beginnings are more about leaving the past behind. Others are more about embracing the future ahead. In any case, a new beginning is a chance to start over again and step up on a new stage.

ADELE: You can stay here. It's your home too.

Excerpt from the play Virgin Tears by Mary Miller

August 12th

Dress Rehearsal

They say that life is not a dress rehearsal ... but in some ways I think they are wrong. I think we are constantly rehearsing, practicing, working to get our parts right. That's the journey of life. It's how we learn. How we move forward. Life may not be a dress rehearsal but it is an ongoing, ever changing, evolving play ... we are the characters and the harder we work to get our parts right the better able we are to take care of our friends, our family, and ourselves.

JOHN: I bet you won Miss Congeniality.

DORIE: Me? Oh no. She was incredible. She had a way of making friends ... getting coffee -- smiling and greeting--always saying you're prettier than she was; and let me tell you, that is one sure fired way to make friends at a beauty pageant contest. Why the night of the finals she came fully equipped with Vaseline for your teeth, double stick tape for your bathing suit, needles, thread, a walking medicine cabinet for headaches and cramps, everything from dental floss to Dr. Scholl's. I voted for her. You can't let that much talent go unrewarded....

Excerpt from the play <u>Light Burgers</u> by Mary Miller

August 13th

Trust

On stage you can always tell the villain, it's the character who says "Trust me!" Now I know that may sound cynical but it seems to be true time and time again. To me trust is not something you declare. It's something you earn, day in and day out, by doing the right thing over and over again.

MASON: What are you afraid of? Trust me.

Excerpt from the play Light Burgers by Mary Miller

August 14th

Nothing to lose.

Before he died (and knowing he was going to die) Steve Jobs gave the commencement address at Stanford University in which he said "remembering you are going to die is the best way I know to avoid the trap of thinking you've got something to lose." It's an amazing thought designed to give you the freedom to pursue, what you feel in your heart, you are destined to do. The freedom to do what you love. What do you have to lose? Some will argue that it depends on who you are and what you have. But the fact of the matter is we come into the world with nothing and we leave with nothing. What we gain and lose in between is pretty much up to us.

Lugano leaned forward and looked at the man she'd known for thirty years. The man she'd worked with for most of her adult life. They had promised to stand by one another long ago, back when nothing was at stake, back when they had nothing to lose.

Excerpt from the book A Matter of Grace by Mary Miller

August 15th

Telephone Operator

Of all the jobs that are never coming back the one I miss the most is the telephone operator. I miss the sound of a real person who was actually interested in answering my call and helping me find an answer. Now given a list of five or six options, none of them good or appropriate, you can spend hours trying to pay a bill, schedule a service, or simply verify an account! As nice as the automotive voice is ... it's not human, and as such, does not think or care what you think. When they say your call is important that's a lie. When they say the call may be recorded you can only wish it was. We have gotten so far away from the meaning of the word service it's doubtful we will ever be able to go back. It's a shame; there are a lot of good people out there who could use the job of being a telephone operator and would be happy to answer your call.

CHANDLER: Hello? HELLO! Mattie? (beat) Adele. (pause) Anyone here?

Excerpt from the play <u>Virgin Tears</u> by Mary Miller

August 16th

The first day ...

Today is the first day of the rest of your life. I remember when I first heard this expression and I thought it was brilliant. I was about ten years old. Now it's become a cliché. But I still find it appropriate on occasion. Because it does mark the beginning of a new day, a new dawn, a chance to get things right. I'm not guaranteeing that will happen but it's a noble goal. It's a reason to get up and try again. No one knows what the day may bring ... why not greet it with open arms ... after all it is the first day of the rest of your life!

ANN: Congratulate me. I did it! Today was the first day.

Excerpt from the play <u>(A Matter of) Grace</u> by Mary Miller

August 17th

Take a Moment

Take a moment to appreciate the stage you are standing on. Take a moment to appreciate the scenery surrounding you. Take a moment to appreciate the people around you. Even if it's not everything you want it to be … be grateful for what it is. Whether it's the end of a long run or the beginning of a new one. Take a moment to appreciate the stage you are standing on.

CHILD: *I won't forget you.*

WOMAN: *I hope that's true.*

Excerpt from the play Take Proper Care by Mary Miller

August 18th

Wardrobe!!

You want to change your life? Start with what you are wearing. If you are wearing the same thing you wore in high school give it a rest! You don't have to throw it away, this isn't about "What Not To Wear," it's finding something "New To Wear." Fall is the perfect time of year to do it. The magazines are full of new looks ... some you wouldn't be caught dead in others you'll be drop dead gorgeous! You don't have to spend a fortune to give yourself a new look ... you just have to take a chance and try something new.

McKenzie wasted little time in discarding her old clothes and upgrading her image with Donna Karen, Ralph Lauren, and Ann Taylor. Her suits were now expensive, tailor-made, and good looking. She liked the way they showed off her figure in a feminine but aggressive manner. She understood the allure of designer clothing and liked the sense of power it gave her.

Excerpt from the book <u>A Matter of Grace</u> by Mary Miller

August 19th

Applause! Applause!

Applause is the sweet sound of success and it's music to anyone's ears! It can come in all shapes and sizes, from a standing ovation to a simple pat on the back. Give it freely. It's the one gift you can't buy for yourself … but you can give it to everyone else.

CLARICE: You're going to be wonderful.

Excerpt from the play <u>Mulberry Lane</u> by Mary Miller

August 20th

Be happy.

I read a passage once that freaked me out. I do this periodically, I randomly open a book, point to a passage, and read it out loud. It's often insightful but rarely mind blowing, except this one time when the passage said: "if you are waiting for someone else to make you happy, you can be waiting your whole life long." Don't wait on happiness to come to you. Go out and get it. Smile. Re-wire your brain for joy. Let go of the past. Make a new memory. Laugh. Be happy!

CHANDLER: It's important to be happy. It's the one thing our parents always wanted us to be. Happy.

Excerpt from the play <u>Virgin Tears</u> by Mary Miller

August 21st

Be young.

Being young is not about looking young or even acting young ... it's about living young! Oliver Wendell Holmes said he would rather be 70 years young than 40 years old. I think I understand what he means. Haven't you ever met a young person who seemed old? Compare that to an old person who seems young? Why not be young ... no matter how old you are?

JANICE: We are not old.

Excerpt from the play <u>Waiting for Oprah</u> by Mary Miller

August 22nd

Be thin.

I have a theory about eating ... it's called the "Three Bite Theory." It goes like this. The first bite of anything is the best. The second bite is good. The third bite is OK. But after that you're simply trying to recreate the sensation in your brain that you had when you ate the first bite. And it's impossible. With each bite the sensation diminishes ... but the calories don't! Why not stop? You've had the best. Remember you can never recreate that first bite ... and sometimes it's not even worth trying.

L.E.: Are you going to eat any of this, Merrillee, or am I going to have to throw it away too!

MERRILLEE: I can't eat. I'm too excited.

Excerpt from the play <u>Light Burgers</u> by Mary Miller

August 23rd

Writing the Dialogue: "Touchdown!"

Every now and then I think it does the body good to throw up your arms and declare touchdown!! You can even dance in the end zone, if you want to, without the risk of a penalty being called. We all deserve to get the ball over the goal line and score a touchdown sometime. It doesn't have to be a momentous occasion. You don't have to catch the Hail Mary pass. Sometimes just getting through the day is reason enough to celebrate. Throw up your arms and yell TOUCHDOWN!

JANICE: Look at Oprah! She came up through the projects and she's made something of her life and I for one would like to say congratulations. You go girlfriend!

Excerpt from the play <u>Waiting for Oprah</u> by Mary Miller

August 24th

Location. Location. Location.

When you find yourself sinking into depression, get up and go for a walk. Walk around the block, around the house, around the room. It doesn't matter where you go ... just move. It's physically impossible to stay depressed when you are in motion. And acting is acting after all. Nobody pays good money to watch someone sit! So get off the couch and go. There is a world of possibility waiting for you outside.

DOWNSTAIRS: (reading from the book) The first person reputed to have "walked around the world." (looking up) You're not planning on walking around the world?! That'll take years!

Excerpt from the play At 3:00 O'clock in the Morning by Mary Miller

August 25th

Believe!

Sometimes you just have to believe in yourself ... whether anyone believes in you or not. A belief in yourself is a gift no one else can give you. They can encourage you and praise you ... but until you believe it yourself nothing else matters. Sometimes you know who you are early in life. Sometimes it takes a lifetime to discover it. But you are worth getting to know ... believe in that.

ANN: And what do you believe?

JOANNE: I believe a mind is a powerful thing, capable of creating anything we need to survive.

Excerpt from the play (A Matter of) Grace by Mary Miller

August 26th

LIGHTS!

One of the key components in any theatrical production is the lighting. I remember being on the set of a film and it was pouring down raining outside. One of those dark, gloomy, don't get out of bed days in New York. But inside, on the set, the stage was lit for a bright sunny day and it made all the difference in my mood, sitting there acting the scene as if the sun was shining. If it's dark in your life turn on the lights both inside your home and inside your mind.

In the dark Margaret watched the twinkling lights on her tiny Christmas tree which stood in the far corner of the room less than four feet away.

Excerpt from the book <u>A Christmas House</u> by Mary Miller

August 27th

Finish this ...

Finishing is as important as starting. In fact I would say finishing is more important, except for the fact that you have to start something to finish it! But so many people begin things and never finish them. Either they get bogged down and lose the energy that propelled them in the first place or they get scared that what they are doing is not worth finishing. But don't be the judge. Anything you begin with a sense of passion is worth seeing through to the end ... just to see what you get!

UPSTAIRS: I quit. I stopped. You were right. It won't count.

DOWNSTAIRS: Hush!

Excerpt from the play <u>At 3:00 O'clock in the Morning</u> by Mary Miller

August 28th

Never let 'em see you sweat!

There is one secret in the theatre that people would do well to take note of in real life and that is when you are on stage and you mess up your lines ... the audience doesn't know it! They don't have clue. They are waiting with baited breath for your every word and as long as you don't turn to them and say: "I screwed up!" ... they'll never know! They'll leave the theatre thinking you were brilliant. Remember you don't have to apologize for what you don't know ... you just have to act with confidence about what you do know ... the audience will never know ... as long as you never let them see you sweat!

CLARICE: George was the only person I ever knew who could make you babble like a schoolgirl. (smiling) And sweat, boy would you sweat.

BERNICE: I did no such thing.

CLARICE: Ice Cream Sunday Social and you're sweating like a pig. (laughing) If I hadn't seen it with my own eyes, I wouldn't have believed it. You should have married him...

Excerpt from the play <u>Mulberry Lane</u> by Mary Miller

August 29ᵗʰ

Experience theatre.

I love a good challenge. Maybe that's why I love theatre. Everything about the theatre should have caused its demise years ago. The idea of getting a group of people together, writing a play, memorizing lines, and acting it out on the stage; while requiring the audience to show up at specific time and pay admission is amazing! Especially these days, when we have the Internet, Facebook, and Twitter. We update, upload, and tweet all day long! There is no escaping the 'real' world ... except at the theatre. And therein lies its magic. It demands something from you. It demands your time and attention. In return you get to experience other people's lives in ways that would be impossible on the Internet, Facebook, or Twitter. You get to experience something that can change your life in ways that the Internet, Facebook, and Twitter never will.

CLARICE: Here it is! Open auditions for their upcoming season. (reading) As You Like It. Romeo & Juliet. Arsenic and Old Lace. Member of the Wedding...

Excerpt from the play Mulberry Lane by Mary Miller

August 30th

Getting to Great

We spend so much of our lives focused on our weakness we forget about out strengths. Now I'm not averse to improving our weakness but when you lead with your strengths you thrive! You can spend hours improving your weakness and get pretty good...but if you spend hours improving your strengths you become great!

LOUISE: We used to be so strong. I looked forward to our meeting everyday of the month. My time with the girls. Away from the kids. Before book club, no one really cared what I thought. So, I didn't think much. Now people ask my opinion and I have one! I'm an intelligent whole human being here.

Excerpt from the play <u>Waiting for Oprah</u> by Mary Miller

August 31st

Once in a Lifetime

When someone wants to get your attention they will say: it's a once in a lifetime offer. Don't bet on it. Offers come around all the time. They come in all shapes and sizes. Most of the time it's just a salesman's pitch to get you to buy something you don't really want. But every now and then when you feel it in your gut you'll know a once in a lifetime offer ... and I suggest you take it. Because every now and then a once in a lifetime offer will be too good to pass up.

The offer the IBM executive had made was fair, fairer than fair, more than she'd ever imagined getting for the old house, and his offer wouldn't be good forever. Abigail had never acted on impulse a day in her life and there she was, sitting bolt upright in the middle of her bed, deciding to sell.

Excerpt from the book A Christmas House by Mary Miller

September 1st

School Calendar

Today is the first day of the new school year. For most teachers this marks the beginning of a new year more than January 1st. I always liked the first day of school. I liked getting my notebooks and pencils and papers together ready for the coming year. I liked going back to school. But then again I was a bit of a nerd! I loved being organized. I still do. I still picture September 1st as the start of a new year with all the possibilities a new year can bring.

WOMAN: You'll start back to school in a couple days, and you'll be so busy you won't have time to think about me.

Excerpt from the play <u>Take Proper Care</u> by Mary Miller

September 2nd

Peace & Quiet

We often say "all we want is a little peace and quiet." That's not necessarily true. At least we don't want it for long. They say the worst punishment you can give a prisoner is to put them in solitary confinement. There is nothing but peace and quiet in solitary confinement and it will drive a person mad. Yes, we want peace and quiet for a little while ... but after a while we crave human companionship. We crave that shared experience. It's one of the reasons theatre has survived, it's an event we share together.

L.E.: (turning to Mason) You know, before you came back this used to be a quiet little town.

MASON: Nothing wrong with a little excitement. Don't you like the feeling of blood rushing through your veins?

Excerpt from the play <u>Light Burgers</u> by Mary Miller

September 3rd

A Good Person

What does it mean to be a good person? I imagine everyone has their own idea ... some more forgiving than others. But in our heart we know what it means to be a good person ... it's just hard to do it all the time! To be a good person you have to think of others before you think of yourself. You have to put their needs ahead of your own. You have to walk a mile in their shoes and look at the world through their eyes. And that's not easy.

FRAN: By the time we got here, he'd forgotten. He wanted to wait in the car. I wanted him to remember so I let him sit there for a while.

MIA: You're a good person.

FRAN: Not so good. I used to get down on my knees. I'd promise to be a better person. Then he wets the bed and I want to kill him and I'm back to square one.

Excerpt from the play <u>Waiting for Oprah</u> by Mary Miller

September 4th

Procrastination

This reminds me of a song ... "procrastination is making me wait." Actually the song is "Anticipation" by Carly Simon ... but today I'm not *anticipating* anything, I'm just putting things off! I have a list of things I should be doing ... and yet I'm watching TV. I don't do that very often but some days I have to take a brake. Ease up on myself and waste a little time. It's OK. I'll never get that time back, but it's OK. You can't run full tilt all the time. It's not healthy! Every now and you have to put your feet up, take a load off, and watch a little TV.

ADELE: Do you ever watch public TV, Mattie?

MATTIE: Some ... but I don't contribute and then I feel guilty so I don't watch much.

Excerpt from the play <u>Virgin Tears</u> by Mary Miller

September 5th

Embrace Change

Do you know the best way to insure your life is a long running production ... embrace change. Embrace change! It's as simple as that. This doesn't mean you have to *like* change, few people do. But if you embrace it instead of fighting it, you'll take the pressure off your heart, your body, and your life. Literally. Fighting change can destroy you. I don't mean you have to blow in the wind with every change imaginable. But if you can adapt to change ... you're more likely to benefit from change. Change happens. There's nothing you can do about it. So embrace it ... look for the good ... and insure yours is a long running show!

LOUISE: *When Oprah comes it's going to change everything.*

ALLISON: *Louise what do you expect is going to happen?*

LOUISE: *Something wonderful.*

Excerpt from the play Waiting for Oprah by Mary Miller

September 6th

Writing the Dialogue: Congratulations!

Congratulations you are a winner! Yes, you are a winner. But wait you say, "I didn't enter any contest." To which I say, "yes you did." You got up, you got out of bed, and you seized the day. Not everyone has that ability and those who do often take it for granted. The ability to breathe, talk, walk, sing, laugh, cry, remember, love, and think! It's amazing how much we take for granted until something happens ... and that's OK. There wouldn't be time enough in the day to do anything if you spent all your time thinking of things you have to be grateful for. But maybe at the end of the day you can take a few minutes to look into the mirror and say "Congratulations" ... you made it through the day.

L.E.: No, it says right here: "Congratulations" Ms. L.E. Jones you are the guaranteed undisputed $5 million dollar winner they've been looking for. They got my name and address and everything. So don't come begging to me when I win the $5,000,000 dollars and the bonus car too boot.

Excerpt from the play Light Burgers by Mary Miller

September 7th

What goes around ...

What goes around ... comes around. You can take that to the bank. I know the expression gets thrown around a lot when we find ourselves caught between a rock and a hard place. When there are no easy answers ... but there's definitely a right one! Sometimes it's more of a wish. Sometimes it's more of a prayer. But if you spread joy, you get joy. If you spread hatred, you get hatred. The Bible calls it reaping what you sow. I call it life. What goes around does come around.

At 3:00 o'clock in the morning defenses are down and tempers flare when a middle-aged accountant, living on the ground floor of an old New York apartment building, finally confronts the neighbor living upstairs who has been walking around in circles overhead for the past 10 hours. Tired and exhausted this downstairs neighbor is determined to put a stop to it now! At 3:00 o'clock in the morning ... what goes around finally comes around.

Excerpt from the play <u>At 3:00 O'clock in the Morning </u>by Mary Miller

September 8th

The show must go on ...

This is true in life and showbiz. The show must go on ... no matter how you feel. An actor has to perform night after night because his audience expects nothing less. They have paid good money and we as actors owe them a good show. It's our job. That's true in life too. No matter how we feel we owe our audience our best, whether they are at work or at home. After all the show must go on ...

MERRILLEE: *I tell you, that was the worst year of my life. I never could go anywhere. I was always waiting for the phone to ring and every morning I had to look my best cause I never knew when I might get that call.*

Excerpt from the play Light Burgers by Mary Miller

September 9th

Chewing the scenery ...

This is an expression we use in theatre when another actor is over acting, upstaging you, and hurting the play. Theatre is not about just one actor, unless of course you are doing a one-person show! They call it dialogue for a reason. In theatre and in life you'll find plenty of these scene-stealing characters. Those who can never stop talking about themselves. Their story is always better, their illness more severe, their experiences grander. They are bores. They bore you and the audience. So if you find yourself losing your audience take a look in the mirror are you chewing the scenery? Pause for a moment and let the other person talk. Your audience will appreciate you more if you relax and give someone else center stage for awhile. You don't have to be the star every day.

WOMAN: She was always taking things of mine. I'm tired of it.

MAN: It won't happen again.

WOMAN: It's not happening now!

Excerpt from the play Patterson's by Mary Miller

September 10th

YouTube Nation

Everyone can now be a star of their own show! No more waiting and anticipating! All you need is a camera and a computer. My how things have changed! It used to cost thousands of dollars and a whole crew to put together a video. Now you can do it yourself in the convenience of your home. There are no more excuses. Now is the time to decide which play you want to live. Re-writing the dialogue. Re-design the stage. Re-cast yourself. It is a YouTube nation. Lights! Camera!! Action!!!

JACKSON: I bought you a video camera.

PEARL: What in God's name for?

JACKSON: To take her picture.

RUTH: Who says I want to have my picture taken.

Excerpt from the play I Witness by Mary Miller

September 11th

World Trade Center

Remember. Recover. Rebuild.

GEORGE: Are you ... all ... all right?

Excerpt from the play <u>Light Burgers</u> by Mary Miller

September 12th

Act Like A Winner: Bio & Resume

When looking for a job (whether on the stage or in life) have your resume ready! It's your calling card. It defines who you are, what you've done, and what you can do. Your bio and resume often tells them more about you than you'll ever have a chance to in person. Make sure it's a good representation of who you are. After all it could make the difference between getting the job or not!

CLARICE: *First, we've got to get you a resume.*

BERNICE: *A resume?! I haven't done anything...*

CLARICE: *Oh, hush. You have too — we'll make it up. Where's your pen. 99% of all the resumes on Broadway were made up at some time.*

Excerpt from the play <u>Mulberry Lane</u> by Mary Miller

September 13th

Act Like A Winner: 30 Second Pitch

You have 30 seconds, starting now, to tell people who you are ... make those 30 seconds count! I don't care whether it's an interview for a job, an audition for a part, or a chance meeting in an elevator with a person who could change your life; you will have 30 seconds to make an impression. Plan, now, on how you want to fill those 30 seconds. Figure out who you are and what you want and write a script. Remember it has to be short, pithy, entertaining, and truthful. It's a tall order, I know, but I'm talking about changing your life. Once it's written ... memorize it ... practice it ... say it to yourself in the mirror ... so when you get the inevitable question: "Tell me something about yourself." You will have an answer. You will be ready. You'll seize the moment and take the stage!

For one solid month McKenzie pitched for a job at the Family Channel.

Excerpt from the book <u>A Matter of Grace</u> by Mary Miller

September 14th

At the Movies

In the movie *The Best Exotic Marigold Hotel* there is a saying that the character Sonny keeps repeating. "Everything will be all right in the end ... if it's not all right ... then it's not the end." I love this idea. It's one of life's lessons I learned from the movie. You see, you can learn a lot at the movies if you take the time to listen.

MERRILLEE: *I remember the movie* <u>*The Day the Earth Stood Still*</u> *the aliens landed in peace but the people shot 'em anyway. My teacher told me it was a metaphor, for our inability to accept anything different, but the aliens still left!*

Excerpt from the play <u>Light Burgers</u> by Mary Miller

September 15th

Get out of the boat!

Joel Osteen once said from the pulpit *"if you want to walk on water...you've got to get out of the boat!"* It struck me then and now as a way of overcoming fear and pursuing a dream. Whatever it is you want it's not going to come to you out of the blue via a knock on the door, a letter in the mail, a call on your cell, an e-mail in your inbox, or a mention on Facebook or Twitter! More often than not you are going to have to go out and get it yourself. Risk failure in order to succeed. There are no guarantees in life ... except for the fact that you'll never walk on water if you don't get out of the boat.

DORIE: Heights. I'm frightened of heights.

JOHN: And you ride a Ferris wheel?

DORIE: On my birthday. My Daddy believed you should do something that frightens you at least once a year. Builds character. Strengthens moral fiber. You ought to try it sometime.

Excerpt from the play <u>Ferris Wheel</u> by Mary Miller

September 16th

Stress Kills

I do believe that stress can kill you! Now, don't start stressing out!! There is a way to deal with it. First notice when you are under stress and step away. Simply walk away. It's the best way I know to defuse a stressful situation. Don't stay and fight. You cannot win. Even when you win ... you lose. I've never seen a situation where anger made it better. For years the experts said to take our stress (and/or anger) out on something like a pillow. Just beat a pillow to death with a bat. However, I found through personal experience, the more I beat that pillow the angrier I got. Yes, I became physically tired and that stopped the actual beating ... but it never stopped the stress. Stress is the gap between where you are and where you want to be ... and you will never get there by swinging a bat.

BERNICE: Clarice, what are you going to do today, besides irritate me?!

CLARICE: I don't know, what do you want to do?

Excerpt from the play <u>Mulberry Lane</u> by Mary Miller

September 17th

Casting Casting

At the beginning of this journal I posed a question: If there was an open casting call to play the part of your life ... would you audition for the role? Would you take the part if you got it? Remember? How does it feel now? Is it any better? Any worse? Have you learned something about yourself and the character you are playing? Look back at your life and see if there are still changes to be made. Miracles can happen ... you just have to believe it is possible.

L.E.: Why are you telling me?

FRANK: I figured you could use a little miracle in your life about now.

Excerpt from the play <u>Light Burgers</u> by Mary Miller

September 18th

Musical Theatre

When writing your own play, why not make it a musical with a full orchestration! No movie would ever be released without a great soundtrack. Why should your life's play be any different? Pick a song you love ... play it in your mind ... sing it out loud ... and see if that song doesn't make a difference in your day.

MERRILLEE: (singing) "Oh I wish I was an Oscar Mayer Wiener ... *that is what I'd truly like to be.e.e... cause if I were an Oscar Mayer Wiener everyone would be in love with me."* I love that song.

Excerpt from the play Light Burgers by Mary Miller

September 19th

Dance to the music.

When writing your musical don't forget to add in the dance numbers too. Everybody loves to dance even if they've got two left feet ... like me! In fact, when I was an actor, on my resume I put "moves well" because I couldn't dance but I could walk across the stage! And I found if you threw in some arm movements it looked choreographed! So pick a tune and dance like no one is watching. Because they're not ... they're dancing too!

BERNICE: I can't .... DANCE!

CLARICE: You can walk can't you?

BERNICE: Of course I can walk!

CLARICE: (writing) "Moves Well"...

Excerpt from the play Mulberry Lane by Mary Miller

September 20th

I'm so excited ...

This weekend I'm going back to New York! I'm so excited!! It's been years since I've been in Manhattan. In fact it's been years since I've been anywhere. My stage has remained so static I fear that I've been walking the floorboards blindfolded. That won't be the case in New York. I'll have to open my eyes, listen closely, and watch where I'm going because my stage will be changing. This weekend why don't you change your stage? Take a trip, get out of the house, or just move the furniture. Change your stage ... it could give you a whole new outlook on life!

MATTIE: (thrilled) You made it! You're here! You're early? I wasn't expecting you until later?

CHANDLER: I took the early bird flight.

MATTIE: You should have let me know. I would have picked you up. Oh, I should have...

CHANDLER: No big deal. I took a cab.

Excerpt from the play <u>Virgin Tears</u> by Mary Miller

September 21st

Today

Today is the tomorrow you worried about yesterday. And if you worry about tomorrow today then you'll be wasting both today and tomorrow! Because with all the worrying we do, we are rarely able to change things. Unless, of course, you are worrying about a problem you can solve ... most of us just worry. Stop! The past is the past and the future is the future. Live today and stop worrying about tomorrow!

MAN: And you decided today would be the day to start?

WOMAN: Otherwise it would be too late.

Excerpt from the play <u>Patterson's</u> by Mary Miller

September 22nd

Love, Loss & What I Wore

I saw this play by Nora Ephron when I was in New York. It was an amazing play. Funny and true. It got me to thinking about how much we focus on the clothes we wear. I remember bell-bottoms and halter-tops. Shirtwaist dresses and cut offs. I remember prom night and New Years Eve. In looking back at some of the outfits I wore they look like costumes from period pieces! If you haven't changed your wardrobe in the last 10 years you might give it a shot. It could make a difference in what happens tomorrow. We've all loved and lost but we don't have to keep wearing the same old outfit.

The lights come up on Robert's backyard. Robert enters, carrying a blanket. He puts the blanket on the ground and lies down, looking up at the stars. Chandler enters. She is now wearing a bright polyester mini skirt-type circa 1980's dress. She carries her bag as she tiptoes in.

Excerpt from the play <u>Virgin Tears</u> by Mary Miller

September 23rd

Narrative Medicine

For several days I was in New York City at Columbia University taking part in a program called Narrative Medicine. A program designed to use *attentive* listening, *close* reading, and *reflective* writing as a means of achieving empathy, understanding, and healing. Based on the idea that everyone has a story and their story has merit Narrative Medicine seeks to recognize that story as a key component to the healing process. A new way of listening, looking, and recognizing the suffering of others in order to create a space when compassion and healing can happen.

DOWNSTAIRS: I can't get it from touching you. (holding out a hand) Put your arm around my neck.

Excerpt from the play At 3:00 O'clock in the Morning by Mary Miller

September 24th

A case for fiction.

In this world where it seems as if only the non-fiction story has value, I'm here to tell you there is more truth in fiction than meets the eye. Fiction is the place where the life imagined and the life lived meet. It is at this crossroads that we find truth. Universal truth. Truth that can guide your own life's story. It is in the fictional character where we find reality ... not only in the world as it is, but as it could be, should be, and can be.

CHANDLER: My father insisted on naming me after Raymond Chandler. Sometimes, I feel like I'm living my life as a fictional character.

Excerpt from the play <u>Virgin Tears</u> by Mary Miller

September 25th

A New Stage

How do you change the stage you are standing on? One of the quickest ways I know is to get out of town. Literally move! I remember when I left the island of Manhattan (I gave up my apartment and shipped my furniture) and moved to St. Simons Island. Talk about two different stages! Both islands are relatively the same size – 12 miles long and 3 miles wide – but that's where the similarities end!

MATTIE: Where are you going?

CHANDLER: (turning to Mattie) Back to Chicago.

MATTIE: I thought you were staying.

Excerpt from the play <u>Virgin Tears</u> by Mary Miller

September 26th

OH, WOW!

At Steve Jobs' eulogy his sister told an amazing story of how his last words were: "Oh, wow! Oh, wow! Oh, wow!" In reading his biography I can tell you he was not a man easily impressed. So I wondered what it was he saw in those last few moments here on earth that caused him to be so excited. A cynical part of me wonders if he planned it? To say it as a last great marketing campaign. The ultimate marketing campaign. But then a less cynical more spiritual side of me wonders what it was he saw? The majesties that lie beyond our reach and understanding. The trick, I think, is to say "Oh, wow" to life as well as death; it is after all an amazing journey we are all on together.

UPSTAIRS: Wow.

Excerpt from the play <u>At 3:00 O'clock in the Morning</u> by Mary Miller

September 27ᵗʰ

What's it worth?

What's it worth? ... is a question that gets bantered about a lot these days. I suppose the answer is in the eyes of the beholder. What something is worth is up to you. Things get bought and sold every day. But what are *you* worth? That's an entirely different question. Try looking at yourself through the eyes of someone else, someone who loves you, and you'll find you're worth a whole lot more than you think.

CHILD: I love you.

Excerpt from the play <u>Take Proper Care</u> by Mary Miller

September 28th

Love yourself!!

I read a short book called *Love Yourself – Like Your Life Depends On It* by Kamal Ravikant. I think it was one of the most important books I've read in a long time. The idea being to love yourself first. (Not unlike putting on the oxygen mask first in an airplane!) But his solution as to how to love yourself was simple. Just say "I love myself" over and over and over again until you do, actually, love yourself in that warm *gooey* way. You don't just "like" yourself, you "love" yourself. The body innately knows what love is and it responds according. It'll improve your health, your mood, and it might help open doors you didn't even know were there. So love yourself like your life depends on it … because it does!

MARGARET: The only bad thing about therapy is that you get in the habit of pouring your heart out to strangers. So you don't think twice about telling your problems to the person sitting next to you on an airplane -- but at home, to your family, where they really might care … you can't say a word.

Excerpt from the play A Christmas House by Mary Miller

September 29th

Resolution

They say we like to watch scary movies because deep down inside we know there will be a resolution. The bad guy will get caught, killed, or run out of town! Good will ultimately prevail. I think that's why people seek out the arts in plays or books or movies. Whether they are mysteries, comedies, or dramas. We want to know how things work out in the end and we are willing to sit through even the most devastating dramas to have that resolution. I think that's the healing part of theatre ... watching to see how the protagonist survives. It gives us hope that we too can survive and there will be a resolution in our own life.

ADELE: I was watching this program about a poor elephant calf, a brand new baby elephant, who wasn't able to walk. His right foot bent under his leg so he could only stand, for a minute, on his ankle and then he'd fall down. The others in the herd had to leave to search for food and water. But his mother wouldn't go.

Excerpt from the play <u>Virgin Tears</u> by Mary Miller

September 30th

Having it all.

People talk about having it all. Some think it's possible, others think it's not. I think it depends on how you define 'all.' Some people think 'all' is everything ... small, medium, and large. Some think 'all' is everyone ... man, woman, and child. I think 'all' is whatever it is you want most. Having it all doesn't necessarily mean you have a boatload of stuff ... it means you have what you want ... and that's having it all.

FRED: We haven't done too bad. We've never wanted for anything.

ABIGAIL: I wanted for you.

FRED: I've got all I want.

Excerpt from the play A Christmas House by Mary Miller

October 1st

A Change of Season

Fall is in the air. Feel it? You can sense a change in the seasons. The air is clean and crisp and cool. The sky is bluer than it is at any other time of the year. Change is happening ... as it does every year at this time. There is something nice about "predictable" change. The change you can count on. The change you look forward to. Seasons come and go. I look on each new season as a new beginning. It's like the opening night of a new show. You can't put your finger on it but you feel it in the air. The electricity is all around you. Take a deep breath ... fall is coming ... and change is possible.

The air was clean and crisp, bringing the landscape of buildings sharply into focus. Ann McKenzie walked down the steps of St. Patrick's Cathedral to the street, but instead of going back to work like she had planned, she turned left and began to walk down 5th Avenue to her home in the Village.

Excerpt from the book <u>A Matter of Grace</u> by Mary Miller

October 2nd

Appreciation

Appreciation is worth its weight in gold. I'm serious. In these times of austerity and deficit a simple "Thank you" can make the difference between feeling needed and feeling used. And, don't kid yourself, there is a huge difference between the two. The difference between being healthy and being sick. Most people who end up in the hospital for stress related illnesses when asked in earnest by their doctor what's wrong? The first thing they often say is I don't feel appreciated. Imagine what a simple "Thank you" can do for the health of your company and home as well as the well-being of your employees and family.

BERNICE: (smiling with gratitude) Thank you.

Excerpt from the play <u>Mulberry Lane</u> by Mary Miller

October 3rd

Sing a song.

I have always said I couldn't write a musical because I don't know enough about music. But it turns out the best way for me to write a musical is to concentrate on the words first. After all lyrics are simply words put to music. I've watched Elton John take random words from a book and create a song. He's a genius! But if you feel like you have a song in your heart ... feel free to make up the words and sing along. It might give you a sense of freedom you've never experienced before.

CLARICE: You want to sing and dance?

Excerpt from the play <u>Mulberry Lane</u> by Mary Miller

October 4th

Better not Bigger

Everyone these days seem to be expounding on the virtues of being big. We are being overwhelmed by bigness. But to my way of thinking big is not always better. We don't need bigger things ... we need *better* things. We don't need bigger ideas ... we need *better* ideas. We don't need bigger ... we need *better*! And that's a big idea worth thinking about.

ABIGAIL: Fred, what is this?!

FRED: (proudly) The kitchen bathroom. It's my idea. People never think to put a bathroom where you really need it.

Excerpt from the play <u>A Christmas House</u> by Mary Miller

October 5th

Upstage/Downstage

Upstage is the location on a stage that is actually furthest away from the audience. (Downstage is the location closest to the audience.) The things that makes the upstage position so powerful is that the person downstage has no ideas what upstage person is doing! It leaves them vulnerable to the whims of other actors and the director. But as powerful as that upstage position is ... I'd rather be downstage ... close to the audience where I can practically reach out and touch them.

DOWNSTAIRS: HELLO! Open Up! Do you hear me?! HELLLOOOO!!!

UPSTAIRS: Who are you?

DOWNSTAIRS: YOUR DOWNSTAIRS NEIGHBOR!

Excerpt from the play <u>At 3:00 O'clock in the Morning</u> by Mary Miller

October 6th

Encore! Encore!

An encore happens at the end of a great show when the audience literally demands that you come back on stage. It's the moment we all live for in theatre and it's a moment we should look for in life. If your audience isn't appreciating you the way you think they should ... maybe it's time to re-evaluate your routine. Shows can get old both on stage and in life. Make sure your routine hasn't become laden with cynicism, sarcasm, and anger. If you find your routine is pushing people away rather than drawing them near ... maybe it's time to re-write your show so your audience will once again beg to see more of you. Encore! Encore!

CLARICE: You're going to be wonderful.

Excerpt from the play <u>Mulberry Lane</u> by Mary Miller

October 7th

Technical Difficulties

In this day and age of modern electronics the one thing we didn't count on when transitioning everything over to the digital revolution is the inevitability of technical difficulties! I don't care how good you are ... how technically advanced you become ... you are always going to be subjected to the fact that every now and then the computer is just going to shut down. Sometimes despite our best efforts the lights won't work, the curtain won't rise, and the computer won't start.

DORIE: Oh my God? What happened?

JOHN: Looks like we stopped.

DORIE: Why?

JOHN: We seem to be stuck.

Excerpt from the play Ferris Wheel by Mary Miller

October 8th

What's your story?

Everyone has a story. Some may be more exciting than others. Some may be more daring. Some more successful. Some more tragic. But everyone has a story. Keep that in mind when you meet people for the first time. Don't be too quick to judge them until you've had a chance to hear their story.

MATTIE: Chandler, you could write something about the Virgin tears. It's the perfect human-interest story.

Excerpt from the play <u>Virgin Tears</u> by Mary Miller

October 9th

Mirror Exercise

In acting class there is an exercise that I think works particularly well both in theatre and in life; it's called the mirror exercise. Two actors stand facing one another and they mirror each others actions. The best thing about this exercise is that it forces you to actually look at your partner. We never really look at people anymore, we always seemed to be distracted by outside forces vying for our attention ... the TV, Internet, Facebook, and Twitter. We're more apt to look at pictures than the real person! At home it's even worse. Today, make a concerted effort to look at the people around you, especially those you love. Things may have changed since the last time you took a really good look.

CHANDLER: It's been a long time, Bobby.

ROBERT: That it has. You look good. You always do.

CHANDLER: (knowing better) Not always.

ROBERT: You always look good to me.

Excerpt from the play Virgin Tears by Mary Miller

October 10th

Act like someone else!

The quickest and easiest way to become the person you want to be is to act like a person you already admire. Pick someone you like (it can be anyone from stage, screen, or life) then for the next 24 hours act like they act. Do what they do ... in thought, word, and deed. See if acting like someone else changes how you would normally respond. We talk a lot about change but we don't know how to do it. Act like someone you like and become the person you want to be.

LOUISE: Allison you are so clever. We should call you Martha.

ALLISON: I'm nothing like Martha Stewart.

LOUISE: No, I mean it in a good way. I still like Martha Stewart.

Excerpt from the play <u>Waiting for Oprah</u> by Mary Miller

October 11th

Now is the time ...

As we get closer to the end of the year people (myself included) begin to think about changes they want to make in their lives in the coming year. Change jobs. Lose weight. You name it! It's easy to sit back and think in a few weeks I will start this, do that, and go there. But what if you started today? Whatever you're thinking of doing then; do it now. You don't have to wait for a certain date, time, or place to make a change. Make that change today and maybe, by the first of the year, that change will be a reality.

CHANDLER: I have to quit my job. Do something else. Get out of there while people still think I'm worth working with, at this rate it's hard to tell who's crazier. Me or my boss.

Excerpt from the play <u>Virgin Tears</u> by Mary Miller

October 12th

Re-think the possibilities.

Every now and then it's a good to stop and re-think the possibilities of what you can do with your life. Fill in the blank: you're never too old to _____? Some of the best artists and writers began their careers late in life. Youth is wonderful but it's often said that youth is wasted on the young! When we're young we are so eager to make our way in the world we sometimes abandon the things we like to do the most. The problem is when we get old we abandon them not because we don't have the time (because we do!) but because we think we can't ... we're too old! Re-think the possibilities; you are never too old to become what you wanted to be when you were young.

MARGARET: I'm fine. Really. I just needed someone to talk to. To help me figure out what I'm doing with my life.

BABS: I thought you were doing what you wanted to do.

MARGARET: I'm doing what I thought I should be doing.

LIZBETH: What do you want to do?

Excerpt from the play A Christmas House by Mary Miller

October 13th

Pollyanna

When I was growing up the name "Pollyanna" was synonymous with naiveté. People who projected a Pollyanna outlook were thought of as simpletons and unsophisticated. The dictionary even defines Pollyanna as a "foolishly or blindly optimistic person." When in actuality Pollyanna was a character in a book written in the early 1900's about a young girl who had a positive outlook on life. Isn't it amazing how we denigrate the positive persona. No wonder it's so difficult to maintain a positive outlook on life, we don't respect it in other people. We don't give them the credit they deserve. It's easy to be pessimistic, the real challenge in life is to be optimistic.

PEARL: What'd he say?

RUTH: He said it be a happy day cause the Lord done let him live another year. He says he's 72 but the way he sees it now he's gonna call himself 27. Figures his numbers are interchangeable now.

PEARL: HUMPH! I don't know who he thinks he's fooling.

RUTH: He ain't fooling anyone, Pearl. He's just trying to get by.

Excerpt from the play <u>Virgin Tears</u> by Mary Miller

October 14th

Good Intentions

Generally speaking when we start a project we begin with the best intentions of finishing it! But sometimes despite our good intentions things go awry. Sometimes real life gets in the way. Sometimes real life is more important. Take time to be with your family and friends whenever you can. Good intentions are great but good friends are better!

MASON: I thought about coming home before. I made reservations. I had every intention of seeing you ...

Excerpt from the play <u>Light Burgers</u> by Mary Miller

October 15th

Recognition

The experts say ... we are all looking for ways to be recognized. But in this day and age it seems we know way too much about people in general and little or nothing about each other personally. With Facebook and Twitter we often post our inner most thoughts but without someone actually there does it matter what we say? I liken it to a tree that falls in the woods ... if no one is there does it make any sound? We are all looking to be recognized but I think the best form of recognition is one-on-one. That moment in time when you look someone in the eye and extend your hand in friendship or love ... that is the recognition we all need to feel whole.

L.E.: I have too looked at Mason.

MERRILLEE: No. Your eyes dart away. You've looked above him, below him, around him. Like my mother used to do me when I died my hair blonde. She never did look me in the eye; she just looked at my hair. Of course she denied it but you can tell when someone is looking you in the eye or the top of your head. (pause) If you ask me Mason is waiting for you to look him in the eye before he can truly be home.

Excerpt from the play Light Burgers by Mary Miller

October 16th

"Everybody is young in heaven."

That's what a good friend of mine said when she miraculously recovered from a ruptured appendix. Virginia Hobson Hicks actually died on the operating table, according to her doctors. Flatlined for over a minute. The thing she remembered, while dead and in heaven she said, was the fact that everyone was young. Even people she remembered as having died in their eighties appeared in their twenties. Their "best-selves" she said and she recognized them all even though she couldn't have known them in their youth. "Everybody is young in heaven." It took the fear of death away and enhanced the joy of living for her and for me.

BERNICE: You're still dead, aren't you.

CLARICE: (quietly) Yes. Three months, two weeks, one or two days ...

BERNICE: ... give or take a few hours. But who's counting?

Excerpt from the play <u>Mulberry Lane</u> by Mary Miller

October 17th

A Good Day's Work

A good day's work means different things to different people. But a good day's work always leaves you with a sense of satisfaction of a job well done, whether you have to come back tomorrow and do the same all over again, or you move on forever. A good day's work leaves you with a feeling of accomplishment. A good day's work is something we should always strive to achieve at the end of every day. Because a good day's work is the real secret to happiness

CHILD: You gonna go work for old lady Brenner?

WOMAN: (stunned) Mrs. Brenner, next door?! What make you think that?

CHILD: She's been asking 'bout you.

Excerpt from the play Take Proper Care by Mary Miller

October 18th

Off the beaten path ...

Every day is froth with possibilities ... you just have to be determined to find them. Sometimes they're right under your nose. Sometimes they feel just out of your reach. But they're always there. Today why not try looking for them in places you wouldn't expect. So often the road we take everyday is so worn we miss the possibilities because we are so familiar with the path. Today, wander off the beaten path and see what you can find.

DORIE: You're not from around here?

JOHN: No. Passing through, saw the wheel and drove on over..

Excerpt from the play Ferris Wheel by Mary Miller

October 19th

One step at a time ...

In theatre there's a saying: to get across the stage you have to take it one step at a time. It's a reminder to stay true to the moment. The trick in theatre, as an actor, is you know how it's going to end because you've memorized the ending! But to play the part you have to forget what you know and live in the moment. I think it's a good idea in life too. So often, we think we know how things will end that we actually drive events to that ending ... good or bad. But if you live in the moment, fully aware of each moment, you may find that the ending you expected is not the ending you get. Practice staying in the moment. Be alive to what's happening now and take the future one step at a time.

DOWNSTAIRS: I hear every step you take! This afternoon I tried to ignore it. At 10:00 o'clock I thought I could sleep through it. By midnight I figured it would stop. But it hasn't and I can't.

UPSTAIRS: I'm just walking.

Excerpt from the play At Three O'clock In The Morning by Mary Miller

October 20th

Secret to Happiness?

The secret to happiness is to love your work. Ironically it doesn't mean you have to love your job, although that would help. But it's OK to not to love your job if it enables you to do the work you love. Understand? Not every play is great … but it's great to be a player. Be proud of the work you do, whatever it is, if it lets you do the work you love. That is the secret to happiness.

JACK: McKenzie even went to church to pray to keep her job. Didn't you, Ann?

(Ann ignores him.)

JOANNE: I don't blame her.

Excerpt from the play (A Matter of) Grace by Mary Miller

October 21ˢᵗ

It's smart to be smart.

It seems today that some people think it's cool to be dumb. Let me tell you, that's the least cool thing you can be! If you are dumb you are destined to sway in the wind on the wings of anyone's opinion. You give up your freedom in ways you cannot imagine. So don't be afraid to learn. Knowledge doesn't have to come from a book ... but it often starts there. Experience alone can be a hard and cruel teacher. Learn from others, from their successes and failures. Learn to read with an open mind, keeping in mind not everything you read will be the truth ... so read a lot. Love to learn. It's smart to be smart.

CHANDLER: (interrupting) Mattie that's crazy.

MATTIE: (upset) It's not crazy!

CHANDLER: It is crazy! I can understand Adele getting upset. But I don't see how a smart, educated, intelligent, young woman like you can stand there and believe or even want a block of wood to cry?!

Excerpt from the play <u>Virgin Tears</u> by Mary Miller

October 22ⁿᵈ

Love means ...

... never having to say anything! ... but wanting to say everything!! Practice saying the words *"I love you"* today, so tomorrow, when you really might need them, the words will be on the tip of your tongue.

ABIGAIL: I love you.

FRED: I know.

Excerpt from the play <u>A Christmas House</u> by Mary Miller

October 23rd

A Good Thing

Most of us think we know a good thing when we see it. The question is how do we find it? I suggest you have the courage to look in places you've never looked before. I know it might sound redundant but I believe that most of us, who say we can't find happiness, are simply looking in the wrong places. We are looking in places we've looked before ... the problem is if you didn't find it there then, trust me, you are not going to find it there now. We have to go out of our comfort zone to find those things that elude our grasp. Get over your fear and look in places you haven't looked before. You may be surprised at what you find.

L.E.: (trying to understand) Merrillee even if that light was a UFO, and it had been calling you, and was going to take you with it; why would you consider going off with some stranger to some place you don't even know?

MERRILLEE: Because I was invited.

Excerpt from the play <u>Light Burgers</u> by Mary Miller

October 24th

Exceeds Expectations

Exceeds expectations is a category that appears on most performance evaluations. It's usually somewhere near the top. But what does it mean? When you exceed someone's expectations you give them more bang for their buck than they expected. In theatre as well as life it's a good thing. It's something we all should strive to achieve. The questions is, however, who's expectations are you exceeding? The people around you? Or your own? To me the only way to determine if you are exceeding expectations is to know, in your heart of hearts, what you expected of yourself.

GEORGE: Look at that! I'll be damn. I didn't know I could do that!

Excerpt from the play Light Burgers by Mary Miller

October 25th

Silence Is Golden

I grew up with the adage *Silence Is Golden* ... but I don't think I ever appreciated it until I got older. There is nothing as soothing, as medicinal, or as healing as silence. Whether you are alone or with a group of people a moment of silence can help calm the nerves and clear your head. In theatre you'll often find the most dramatic moment on stage is when the characters are not talking! Keep this in mind ... when you find yourself at a loss for words ... stop talking! Maybe the best response is silence, after all silence is golden.

JOHN: STOP! I'll pay you a hundred dollars if you don't say another word!

Excerpt from the play Ferris Wheel by Mary Miller

October 26th

Promises, Promises

Have you ever promised more than you could deliver? It happens all the time. It's a hard lesson to learn. There is a fine line between being optimistic and being wrong! Sometimes you can be optimistic and wrong at the same time. But my rule of thumb is to promise what you think you can ... work like hell to make it happen ... and never stop trying to do more. That's a promise to yourself that I promise you is a promise worth keeping.

MATTIE: You won't be sorry. I promise.

Excerpt from the play <u>Virgin Tears</u> by Mary Miller

October 27th

Turn away.

Sometimes the best thing we can do when we are confronted with things we can't change is to simply turn away. You do not have to fight every battle. Sometimes it's best to step back and see how much energy, anxiety, stress, and sleepless nights it's going to cost you if you do engage. Sometimes the cost is not worth the effort. Even if you are right! Even if you win!! Learn to turn away and live to fight another day. A day when the battle might really be worth winning.

ANN: I have no intention of fighting Joanne.

HUGH: She's a bitch.

ANN: But I never should have said it.

Excerpt from the play (A Matter of) Grace by Mary Miller

October 28th

Time Traveler

Have you ever felt like you've been here before? They call it deja vu and it can happen at the oddest places. Suddenly (in an unfamiliar place) you're struck with the undeniable sensation that you've been here before. Well, I believe you have! At least you might have? Think about it. We are all just a mass of molecules ... right? And according to Einstein matter cannot be created or destroyed. So ... some of the matter that is in you has, in fact, been here before. When you get that deja-vu feeling take a special note to look around. There may be clues there that can help you in your life ... after all who's to say you're not a time traveler too!

MERRILLEE: Maybe when I get back I'll be younger than I was when I left. You know space travel is different than cross country.

Excerpt from the play <u>Light Burgers</u> by Mary Miller

October 29th

Fool me once ...

Fool me once ... shame on you. Fool me twice ... shame on me! It's an important lesson to learn. But you don't always have to learn from experience. Theatre is a great teacher! All you have to do is sit back and watch. Yes, they are actors, but their problems are real. There's no need to go through everything yourself ... watch and learn. So, fool you once? ... I doubt it!

GEORGE: I don't care what "the light" wants. I am not gonna stand there like some fool - looking up saying: "Where? Where?" I know a good thing when I see it ... whether I see it or not!

Excerpt from the play <u>Light Burgers</u> by Mary Miller

October 30th

Competition

Some say that competition is a bad thing ... but I'm a firm believer that competition can be a good thing. It can be the driving force that helps us achieve things beyond our means. It can be a motivating factor that gets us out of bed in the morning or off the couch in the evening. Whether it's in sports or school or theatre or even just with yourself ... competition can bring out the best in you. Even if you lose! You can always say you tried. So engage in a little friendly competition and see how far you can go!

DOWNSTAIRS: Oh for heaven's sakes ... (rethinking the argument) ... then if you have to break a record, do you have to break one that bothers me?! Can't you do something else. Something quieter? (flipping through the book, looking at different entries) Why not - "Beer Coaster Flipping" - it's simple, quiet. You still get your name in print. That is the point, isn't it? What difference does it make what you do? He only flipped 102 coasters.

Excerpt from the play <u>At Three O'clock In The Morning</u> by Mary Miller

October 31st

Halloween

It's the scariest time of the year! It's the only time of year when we are actually encouraged to dress up in a costume and pretend to be something we are not. Of course being Halloween those costumes are usually demons, ghosts, and goblins. Not my favorite things! But what if you took the spirit of Halloween and dressed up as something you'd really like to be. It may not be scary, but, trust me, the reward will be sweeter than any candy you'll get as a goblin!

CLARICE: When you get out there treat yourself to a new outfit. Promise me you won't pull anything out of those old garbage bags!!

Excerpt from the play <u>Mulberry Lane</u> by Mary Miller

November 1st

Research

I don't care what business you are in or what you do for a living the first thing you should do before doing anything new is research. Look at both the positive and negative sides of any venture you are considering. It's easier to do today than in any other time in our history because sources like Google let you research without ever leaving the comforts of your own home! This isn't to say don't be spontaneous. But being blindly spontaneous is a recipe for disaster. Take time to research ... and remember any offer that has to be acted upon immediately is an offer you should step away from ... immediately!

GEORGE: Last night Mason and I went around and put up flyers all over town announcing ..."Tonight Is The Night".

FRANK: The night for what?

GEORGE: The LANDING OF THE LIGHT ... tonight that light is going to land right outside on my front lawn.

L.E.: (reading the flyer) Oh, for crying out loud! You said that?! Mason encouraged you to do this? No wonder we haven't had anyone in here all day - scared to death they'll be sitting here and some "UFO" is gonna land in their laps.

Excerpt from the play <u>Light Burgers</u> by Mary Miller

November 2nd

Moving On

In life as in theatre people come and go. They are not just passing acquaintances they are people who mean something to you in your life. We think, in the moment, we will always be together and then the moment passes and things change and people move on. Let them go. You cannot hold on to the past. Remember them fondly and open your heart to those people who are here now ... standing right in front of you.

WOMAN: I'm gonna miss her. Do you think she knows that?

MAN: I imagine.

WOMAN: Do you think she's looking down on us now?

MAN: No. I don't think she's studying us.

Excerpt from the play Patterson's by Mary Miller

November 3rd

Class Picture

An old friend of mine sent me a picture of my nursery school class. It struck me how much I've changed in some ways and how little I've changed in other ways. My hair is no longer black. I no longer wear smock dresses; but the way I held my hands together anxiously awaiting the shot is something that I recognize in pictures taken today! My friend asked me to note what I *used* to remember about growing up in Atlanta. First thought was Atlanta used to be a small town. I used to shop at Lenox mall except when it rained because malls weren't enclosed back then! I used to ride the Pink Pig at Rich's department store. I used to drink Coca-Cola from a glass bottle. Atlanta used to be the place where I lived. It used to be a stage I knew well. It's been a long time since those days in Atlanta. I can only return to that stage in my mind and yet the memories are still strong and vibrant and alive. But that's not the stage I'm on now. I think it's interesting to note how often we transition from stage to stage. Life and theater are alike in that way. You can step off or on to any stage you want. Find an old picture; ask yourself how much you've changed. Then ask yourself if it's for better or worse ... and realize you can change the stage you are on and make a whole new picture for yourself and your life.

FRANK: What 'little' things have you got in here?!

MERRILLEE: I got pictures .of me and my family and my family's family to show where I come from. I got a snow globe of a Peach Blossom from when we lived in Atlanta. My blue ribbons, a bag full of hair rollers, and a jar full of dirt from the backyard of the house I grew up in.

Excerpt from the play <u>Light Burgers</u> by Mary Miller

November 4th

I'm sick.

More often than not I'm able to stay well, just by acting healthy! But every now and then I get hit and, like it or not, I have to admit I'm sick. It's never fun. It's always tiring. And it can be down right aggravating. But, like it or not, sometimes the human body just stops and tells us it's time to slow down. Take time. Life is a marathon not a sprint! Take time for your health!! Sometimes the best way to act healthy is to stop acting and get a good nights sleep.

DOWNSTAIRS: Are you sick?

UPSTAIRS: (limping, protecting the right knee) I'm fine.

DOWNSTAIRS: If you're sick, you should go to bed!

Excerpt from the play At Three O'clock In The Morning by Mary Miller

November 5th

Think and Grow Rich

Think and Grow Rich is a book written by Napoleon Hill back in the 1930's but it's well worth a read today. It talks about coming out of The Depression and making a rich life for yourself. Of course he was talking about The Great Depression of 1930's ... but I'm talking about *the great depression* that can come over your mind at any time. Napoleon Hill bases much of his philosophy on the power of the mind and the imagination to achieve anything you want in life. "You are only limited by the limits you place on yourself." That is a philosophy that was true then and is true now.

JACKSON: (explaining) Look, on my way home I got to thinking .... maybe it wasn't just an accident that that video camera was the first thing I saw. Maybe the Lord put that camera in front of me for a reason. And then it come to me ... you know how I'm so good with my hands. How I can fix anything. Well, I got to thinking that I could get you to video tape me while I'm working – fixing a car or something – and I could explain it all ... all that I'm doing while I'm doing it. Then I could sell that tape as a ... instructional video tape. You know. Or rent it. To people who don't know nothing about fixing cars. And I wouldn't stop with just cars, I could fix radios and TVs and ...

Excerpt from the play I Witness by Mary Miller

November 6th

Act like a winner.

The best advice I can give to anyone at any stage in life is to always and I mean always act like a winner. This does not mean going around bragging about all you have accomplished. It means embracing the personality of a winner. Being positive, upbeat, eager, enthusiastic, and willing. These are characteristics that will win you both friends and opportunities. How do you act like a winner? The first step is to stand up straight and smile!

CLARICE: Stand up, Bernice, how tall are you?

Excerpt from the play <u>Mulberry Lane</u> by Mary Miller

November 7th

Acting is Believing

Truly great actors believe in their parts so much they actually convince you they are who they say they are! How do they do this? By becoming the greatest salespeople on earth. You see, they not only have to sell it to you ... they first have to sell it to themselves.

MATTIE: You know Adele. She's so sure! She can convince anyone. And when you're sitting here, waiting, I promise you can feel something in the air.

Excerpt from the play <u>Virgin Tears</u> by Mary Miller

November 8th

Act Again … Now

Remember when we started I said if you want something to happen … act like it has already happened.? It was true then and it's true now. If you want to be thin … act thin now! If you want to be happy … act happy now! There is something exciting about doing it *now* that empowers you and propels you forward. So, if you didn't act then … act now!

WOMAN: If I don't do something now I'll never get another chance to prove I can.

Excerpt from the play <u>Patterson's</u> by Mary Miller

November 9th

Better than Gold

A good idea is worth more than gold ... because a good idea can take you anywhere you want to go. Be on the look out for good ideas. They can hit you anytime day or night. Once you start acting on them you'll find they come quicker and quicker. Every great thing started as a good idea. Don't let other people discourage you. Act on that good idea you've had tucked away in the back of your mind and see where it might lead you. If it was a good idea to you, chances are it'll be a good idea to someone else!

PEARL: That wasn't a bad idea Jackson had 'bout that camera. (pause) The more I think about it ... it wasn't a bad idea.

Excerpt from the play I Witness by Mary Miller

November 10th

Burning Passion

Have you ever asked yourself why things are possible for some people and impossible for others? Is it luck? I don't think so. Is it fortune? Money helps but it's not always the answer. Is it connections? Sure but they can only take you so far. Is it hard work? Sometimes but not always. I think the only sure path to success is passion. A burning desire to succeed. Successful people have a vision of what is possible and the passion to make it happen.

DOWNSTAIRS: You're crazy. You'll kill yourself in the process and then where will you be?

UPSTAIRS: In the record book.

Excerpt from the play At Three O'clock In The Morning by Mary Miller

November 11th

The obstruction that propels us!

Often in life we let the thing that blocks us ... stop us from achieving our goals. But chances are when you are blocked you have to work harder, think clearer, and dream bigger. So, why not change your point of view and try looking at those obstacles as opportunities to propel you forward in new directions you might never have discovered if you hadn't been blocked in the first place? I've said it before but I'll say it again that person, place, or thing that looks like a rock ... use them as a stepping stone to reach up higher!

GEORGE: I'm going to fill in that ditch so it's clear just where my property begins and the city's ends!

L.E.: George you are not going to turn this place into one great big mud puddle!

GEORGE: I don't want this place to go under.

MASON: You aren't going to do anything but make it harder for those people who want to eat here to get here.

GEORGE: They can come through. Those that want to.

Excerpt from the play <u>Light Burgers</u> by Mary Miller

November 12th

Buying Happiness

They say you can't buy happiness but I disagree. You may not be able to buy happiness for yourself, but you sure can buy happiness for someone else. Now I'm not advocating sending money in the mail to family members (or friends) in an effort to buy their love ... although it could help. But I am advocating reaching out and giving someone in need a helping hand. You don't have to look very far. Some call it charity others call it volunteer work. I just call it a good deed. Look for ways to make someone else happy and you will be happy yourself. Yes, you can buy happiness if you spend it on someone else.

L.E.: Have you got any money?

MERRILLEE: I don't need money.

L.E.: I've got money.

Excerpt from the play <u>Light Burgers</u> by Mary Miller

November 13th

A Broken Heart

Every now and then your heart is going to get broken ... no matter what you do. It happens. It takes the wind out of your sails and the kick out of your step. But don't let it keep you down for too long. After all the only way to have a broken heart is to put your heart out there. To take a chance. And that's a good thing. Give yourself time to heal. But not too much time. The best thing to do for a broken heart is to pick it up, dust it off, and get back in the game.

MERRILLEE: You know I think there might be some connection. With the light shining and Mason coming back.

L.E.: I don't think they have anything to do with one another.

MERRILLEE: You haven't looked at the light and you haven't looked at Mason. That's hardly a coincidence you can ignore.

Excerpt from the play Light Burgers by Mary Miller

November 14th

What did you say?

Words come and go today at the speed of light. They are abbreviated, edited, and condensed into symbols and letters that appear more like secret code than actual words. It doesn't mean words have disappeared, but they have been replaced with a different type of communication. But no matter how they are written, words still matter. A thumbs up or thumbs down says success or failure in any language. The thing that is different today is that words don't disappear like they used to when written on paper ... words written in Facebook or Twitter can have a life of their own in cyberspace. They can follow you for years and years ... for better or worse. So, be careful what you say ...

CLARICE: That's a bold face lie! You take it back!!

Excerpt from the play <u>Mulberry Lane</u> by Mary Miller

November 15th

What is important?

What's important in your life? Ask yourself. It's a question worth pondering. Seriously. Quietly. In the privacy of your own mind. Sometimes the answer will surprise you. Sometimes you'll find it's not what you thought it was. Sometimes it's not all the stuff that you've accumulated or the awards you have won. Sometimes it's not even the people you have in your life that you love and can count, although they do have a great deal of value and importance. But I'm talking about you and your life. What is important to you? It's a question worth answering.

FRAN: Is it that important to you?

LOUISE: Yes.

Excerpt from the play <u>Waiting for Oprah</u> by Mary Miller

November 16th

A world of ideas.

If it's true that matter can neither be created or destroyed (a fact well know in the scientific world.) Then what about thoughts and ideas? What happens to ideas when great thinkers and writers die? Do their ideas die with them? Or do those ideas still exist somewhere in the universe waiting for the next great thinker or writer? After all, where does a good idea come from? Your brain? Yes. But before that ... does that idea exist ... or is it created when you think of it? I don't know. I just know that I've experienced that moment of euphoria when the perfect idea pops into my head so many times that now I have begun to trust it. Believe it. Expect it. Ask for it! Tonight before going to bed put a call out to the universe and sleep with a pen by your bed and expect an answer by morning.

MERRILLEE: It was like sharing a personal secret with someone without having to tell it to anybody. It took a weight off my shoulders and I cried like a baby standing there talking to this stranger in the light.

Excerpt from the play <u>Light Burgers</u> by Mary Miller

November 17th

The physical act of writing.

There is something different that happens in the brain when you physically write a word as opposed to typing and texting ... and that is the physical connection between your body and your mind. A connection a computer can only mimic. The physical act of writing is more intense, more intimate, and more immediate. The physical act of writing makes whatever you write real. Real joy. Real pain. Real anger. Real love. To actually feel the word as you write it makes you more aware of what you are saying and gives it a life of its own. Give yourself time to actually write your thoughts down. Pick up a pen and paper and discover what you really think.

ADULT CHILD: (V.O.) August 12, 1955. I remember. I kept a five-year diary that year. It was a birthday present I opened early ... two months before I turned ten. In 1955 Eddie Fisher married Debbie Reynolds. Rosa Parks refused to ride in the back of the bus and Bill Haley and the Comets sang "Rock Around the Clock". We shared a lot of things that year, she and I. Nehi Sodas, Moonpies, Davy Crockett "Coonskin" caps, the Mickey Mouse Club ... and the death of my parents.

Excerpt from the play Take Proper Care by Mary Miller

November 18th

Don't wait!!

Today there is often a feeling of being able to wait, a sense that there is plenty of time. After all we are all living longer healthier lives. Surely there is no pressure to do everything now. But there is! That's what I'm here to tell you. Don't waste time waiting … no matter what you are waiting for. Go out there and meet it half-way at the very least. Go! Test yourself. Meet new people. Experience new things. Whether you are twenty or sixty life begins now!!!

MERRILLEE: You are welcome to come with me.

L.E.: Right! Just pick up and go off into outer space with little green men.

MERRILLEE: They are not green. That is a common misnomer.

Excerpt from the play <u>Light Burgers</u> by Mary Miller

November 19th

Small, Medium, Large

In the world of retail things are categorized as small, medium, and large. It's a great way to organize your life too. Consider this … when faced with a problem why not decide whether it's small, medium, or large. Then you know exactly the firepower it's going to take to solve it! You can arm yourself for the battle ahead … whether it's small, medium, or large.

JANICE: We should have warning signals in a relationship. Yellow–Calm. Orange–Danger. Red–Alert. Give us some clues as to what to expect next. Prepare yourself – put the gas masks on and load the weapons.

Excerpt from the play <u>Waiting for Oprah</u> by Mary Miller

November 20ᵗʰ

Ready, Set, Go!

The first key to success is to be ready. To be in a mind frame to see it on the horizon and be able to move at a moments notice. The second key to success is to be set. Don't let anyone knock you over with words or actions. So, take your rightful place, keep your goal in mind, plan a course of action, and then GO!

MERRILLEE: HERE I AM! I'M READY!! Take me NOW!!!

Excerpt from the play <u>Light Burgers</u> by Mary Miller

November 21st

Win, Lose, Draw

The outcome shouldn't really matter … the fact of the matter is you got into the game! So many times people sit on the sidelines of life and watch it go by. Life is not a spectator sport. To be involved you have to get involved. It doesn't matter how or where. Your stage can be as big or as small as you want. The fact is win, lose, or draw you'll never know what you can do until you try.

MERRILLEE: (proudly) I was the third runner-up. You know, if the reigning Miss USA was unable to fulfill her duties and the first runner-up was unable to fill hers and the second runner-up was unable, I would have had to do it.

Excerpt from the play <u>Light Burgers</u> by Mary Miller

November 22nd

Group Photo

At the start of every show there is a tradition we observe in the theatre and that's the cast photo. Everyone, fully dressed in costumes, stands on the stage and they take a picture. That picture is used to market the play in newspapers, magazines, and in the playbill itself. But to me the best thing about the group photo is that it preserves the moment. The moment in time before the run of the show when everything thing is possible!

MATTIE: All we have to do is set up Adele's camera to automatic and photograph the three of us, sitting right here.

Excerpt from the play <u>Virgin Tears</u> by Mary Miller

November 23rd

Obsessive Compulsive

Over the course of the past year I've given pause on more than one occasion to wonder if this day-by-day journal could be an obsessive compulsion? To attempt to write something like this day after day has been daunting! A challenge to say the least. Some days have been better than others. But most days it's been a labor of love ... because most days I discover something new about Acting Healthy that I hadn't thought of the day before. Each day I surprise myself with the ability to come up with something different. If that's obsessive compulsive ... it's a virtue in this case.

DOWNSTAIRS: You've been walking around for hours!

UPSTAIRS: So?

Excerpt from the play At Three O'clock In The Morning by Mary Miller

November 24th

Hidden Secrets

Sometimes the best secrets are hidden secrets. That may sound like a misnomer, after all, most secrets are designed to be concealed. But the secrets I'm talking about are *secrets* that are designed to be found! Books are full of hidden secrets. Plays are based on hidden secrets. We often live our lives with hidden secrets … hoping someone will take the time to find us.

WOMAN: Now wait. What are you fixen to do?

CHILD: You'll see. Start counting when I get to the top of the stairs. OK?

Excerpt from the play <u>Take Proper Care</u> by Mary Miller

November 25ᵗʰ

The First Step

The first step is the most important step to make … because it's often the hardest step to take. The first step is the beginning of an undetermined journey. The first step is the scariest because it starts on unfamiliar territory. The first step is the first thing you have to do to change your life. The first step to being healthy is … Acting Healthy.

JOAN: This is my first time.

BARBARA: (stunned) You're kidding.

Excerpt from the play NEXT by Mary Miller

November 26th

Out of Town Run

One thing everyone can learn from theatre is the advantage of having an out of town run. This is a run of the show … away from the harsh lights of Broadway to work out the kinks and errors before making that grand debut. It's a good practice to keep in mind before you attempt to do anything important. Practice it in front of the mirror. Test it out on your friends. Whether it's a job interview, a speech, or meeting your new in-laws! Practice what you're going to say before the event. Have an out of town run so your opening night can be a smash!!

CHANDLER: I'm just trying to figure out what I'm going to say to Robert.

MATTIE: And what are you going to say?

CHANDLER: I don't know. I thought if I said it out loud, I'd stumble on an answer.

Excerpt from the play <u>Virgin Tears</u> by Mary Miller

November 27th

Time to be Thankful

Gratitude is one of the most powerful emotions in the world. Being grateful is a state of being that fills your heart and soul with love and empathy. It's the gateway to compassion. It's a humbling feeling when you own up to the fact that you cannot do everything alone. We all need help. As the years go on I get more and more grateful. Grateful for my health, my family, and my friends!

FRAN: I used to pray for that big miracle ... that sweeping miracle that would take all this away. Now I pray for small miracles ... that brief moment of recognition when George is himself for however short a time that is. (She hands her name tag to Louise) Oprah gave me that moment. If she walked through that door this minute she couldn't do anymore for me and I'm grateful. Will you tell her thanks?

Excerpt from the play <u>Waiting for Oprah</u> by Mary Miller

November 28th

Sales, Sales, Sales

This is the time of year everyone pulls out their credit cards (and cash!) and heads for the malls!! It's a crazy time of year. Packed with holiday shoppers of all ages and sizes ... shopping (usually) for people other than themselves! That's the magic of the holiday season. For the next few weeks everyone will be thinking, not just of themselves, but of the people they love. And if you ask me this is the beginning of the best time of year.

ABIGAIL: It was my Christmas present to your Father. Merry Christmas, Fred!

Excerpt from the play <u>A Christmas House</u> by Mary Miller

November 29th

Finding Time

This is also the busiest time of year! It's almost overwhelming. But the thing I keep in mind, when I don't think I have time, is to break up the day into three eight hour shifts. Eight hours for sleep. Eight hours for work. Eight hours for me. Somehow when I break the day up like that I set boundaries on my time and I don't waste it as much. Give yourself eight hours to sleep. Eight hours to work. Eight hours for yourself. That might be all the time you need!

CHILD: (stalling) You think we got time to go down to Mr. Moore's Texaco gasoline station. I sure would like a moonpie and a grape Nehi before I go.

Excerpt from the play Take Proper Care by Mary Miller

November 30th

Breathe

Don't forget to breathe! Do it now!! Take a deep breath. It may be a while before you have a chance to take another. As much as I am a firm believer in embracing life to the fullest, there is wisdom in taking a moment to gather your strength. We cannot run full tilt all the time. On stage it would be exhausting for the actors and the audience. So today stop what you are doing and breathe!

JOHN: Just take a deep breath. It's mind over matter. Just breathe. Breathe.

Excerpt from the play <u>Ferris Wheel</u> by Mary Miller

December 1st

Magical time of year...

Call me sentimental but I love Christmas. I love the decorations. I love the music. I love the feeling that comes over people when they are buying gifts for someone else other than themselves. It's a magical time of year. Take time to notice it and appreciate it. For the next 30 days smile first at the people you see at the mall, in the office, at home, or in line! Chances are they'll smile back! Tis the season!!

BABS: I love Christmas! I love Christmas!!

Excerpt from the play A Christmas House by Mary Miller

December 2nd

Quitting is not an option.

I say this not to put pressure on you (or me!) ... I say it because it's true. The key to success, any success, is finishing what you started. I know along the way we are apt to judge ourselves. We think what we are doing is not worth it, not good enough, or just plain bad! But that's not true. It's just not finished. So before you judge anything ... finish it first. When you do, you'll probably find in retrospect, that it's much better than you imagined it would be when you were stuck in the middle. Quitting is not always an option.

DOWNSTAIRS: What do you mean you can't stop!

Excerpt from the play <u>At Three O'clock In The Morning</u> by Mary Miller

December 3ʳᵈ

The right words.

Finding the right words is not easy, whether you are writing a tweet or a best selling novel. After all, if words were all it took to make a best seller ... the dictionary would be the best selling book in the world!! But words are nothing without feelings. So, when you are stumped to find the right words, look in your heart. That's where they'll be one after the other.

"Love you," he said. Howard was a man of few words. He didn't talk much but what he said counted.

Excerpt from the book <u>A Christmas House</u> by Mary Miller

December 4th

One-Day Sale

This holiday season have you noticed that everyday seems to be a one-day sale? Then, when that day comes and goes, the next day is another one-day sale? And then the next, and the next, and the next?! When I first started noticing this I felt like it was false advertising. Then I got into the spirit and realized, yes, everyday is a one-day sale, because everyday you wake up is a gift. How quickly we forget this. So, get out there and enjoy the day. Think of it as a one-day sale and make the most of it!

"Fred, what is a tub doing in here? Who ever heard of putting a tub in a bathroom like this?" Abigail asked as she looked at the tub in the unfinished kitchen bathroom. "They were on sale!" Fred replied. "And I know how much you hate to take showers, so I thought, why not!" He proudly sat on the edge of the white porcelain tub.

Excerpt from the book <u>A Christmas House</u> by Mary Miller

December 5th

A cliché is a cliché.

People often criticize others for speaking or writing in clichés, but let me tell you, a cliché is only a cliché because it is true. Something that was true yesterday, is true today, and will be true tomorrow is a cliché! There is no getting around it. But the truth is not always easy. Sometimes it's the hardest thing in the world. So, cliché or not, be true to yourself ... it's the greatest cliché of them all.

JOHN: Truth is stranger than fiction.

Excerpt from the play <u>Ferris Wheel</u> by Mary Miller

December 6th

It takes time.

Everything we do in life takes time. Some things take less time than others. Some things take more time than you expected. But everything takes time. It's important to remember this, particularly now, when everyone is hustling and bustling about trying to get a list of things done before the end of the holidays. Just remember everything takes time.

FRED: Abby, building a house takes time.

Excerpt from the play <u>A Christmas House</u> by Mary Miller

December 7th

Coming home.

In December people think more about coming home than any other time of the year. Home is where the heart is during the holidays for better or worse!! As much as we hope and pray that the holidays are a happy and joyous occasion, they can be stressful. Feelings can get hurt. Tempers flare. We have tremendous expectations driven by television and the movies to have a Merry Christmas! That's not always possible. Going home can be difficult even in the best of circumstances. This year try to make room in your life for all the members of your family to come back home ... whether they are miles away or standing right in front of you.

L.E.: Mason, why are you here?

MASON: Dillard is my home.

Excerpt from the play <u>Light Burgers</u> by Mary Miller

December 8th

Joy to the World

If you listen closely you'll notice that the music around us has changed. Everywhere you go you hear the sounds of Christmas. Even the most popular musicians have their take on the holiday classics. It's a tradition. It's amazing when you think about it. The entire soundtrack of our life has changed to one of hope, peace, love, and joy!

As they worked, the three sisters sang "We Three Kings" of Orient are ... making up the words as they decorated the house for Christmas.

Excerpt from the book <u>A Christmas House</u> by Mary Miller

December 9th

Calm before the storm ...

Often the expression the "calm before the storm" is used as a negative, that brief moment before an upcoming disaster that people dread. But sometimes the calm is just that ... a moment of peace and reflection before we get on with the business of life. A moment to revive and renew. A moment to reflect and give thanks. A moment that is often overlooked in our rush to the future. Take time today to rest in the peace of the moment ... before the rush of the holiday season.

Abigail had never acted on impulse a day in her life and there she was, sitting bolt upright in the middle of her bed, deciding to sell their old home. It was to be her Christmas present to Fred. Leaving her life and entering his ... a gift she thought - what a wonderful gift!

Excerpt from the book A Christmas House by Mary Miller

December 10th

Barbara Walters Special

Barbara Walters once interviewed Robin Roberts from *Good Morning America* as one of The Most Fascinating People Of The Year for having survived an extremely rare bout with cancer and doing it on the air! But as courageous as that was the thing that impressed me most about Robin was her outlook on life. She said if she found herself depressed it was because she was living in the past. If she was anxious, she was living in the future. When she was happy, she was living in the moment. Never have I heard the value of "living in the moment" be so clearly articulated.

PEARL: It's your world now ... yours and Ruth's. I can't do any more. I done gone and got confused between the past and the present and they ain't got nothing to do with one another – nothing at all.

Excerpt from the play I Witness by Mary Miller

December 11th

Chance encounter.

Some days you get up and start in one direction and for whatever reason you end up going in another. Some days just can't be planned ... for better or worse! Maybe these days are the best days. Because on these days (the ones you don't plan!) you never know who you might run into and those chance encounters could make all the difference in the world.

JOHN: I would have taken another seat but the line is too long to let anyone ride by themselves ... (awkward pause) ... They force you to be a couple whether you want to or not ... not that I mind. I mean it's a pleasure.

Excerpt from the play Ferris Wheel by Mary Miller

December 12th

What goes around.

They say that what goes around comes around. In some circles it's called karma. In others it's called justice. I can't say for sure which camp I fall into but I do believe it's true. At least I hope it is. Sometimes people can be so mean it's hard to believe they can sleep at night. Others can be so kind it's hard to believe they grew up in these times of anger and violence. Me? I just try to do the best I can because I was raised to believe what goes around ... comes around!

WOMAN: Child, you gots to love me so much that the only color you see is the color of my heart. And I got to love you the same. And we got to take proper care to treat people right, that's the only way we be able to live together ... you and me and Mary Lou O'Callahan ...

Excerpt from the play Take Proper Care by Mary Miller

December 13th

Two for One

It's the holidays and everywhere you look you see sales 10%, 20%, 30%, 40% off and more! But the best deal of all is "two for one." Just imagine if you could get "two for one" everyday!! We could get something for ourselves and give something to a friend. Of course this isn't possible. Stores would quickly go into bankruptcy. But there is one thing that's always guaranteed two for one and that's a smile. Give a smile and you'll get a smile. It may be corny but it's true!

JACKSON: I see it! I see a smile ... you can't fool me. I see it.

Excerpt from the play <u>I Witness</u> by Mary Miller

December 14th

Sadness too.

'Tis the season to be jolly, but it's also the season to be sad. Sad for what was ... what could've been ... and what will never be. Sad for those family and friends who are here and those who are gone. Christmas is a season of mixed blessings. So be aware during the holiday season that not everyone is as happy as they'd like to be and bring them into your life and spread a little joy ... because with the season there is sadness too.

LIZBETH: Don't cry, Momma, it's Christmas.

Excerpt from the play <u>A Christmas House</u> by Mary Miller

December 15th

Now or Never

If there is anything you meant to do this year that you haven't done, I suggest you get busy doing it! It's now or never ... at least for this year.!

ALLISON: *Well, now that you mention it.*

Excerpt from the play <u>Waiting for Oprah</u> by Mary Miller

December 16th

A cold wind blowing!

If you've ever experienced the beach in winter you'll know how cold it gets. I think it's because of the water ... the moisture chills you to the bone. But whether you are down south or up north, when a cold wind blows it's best to batten down the hatches, stay inside, light a fire, and read a book (or a play!) Take time for yourself because it's the perfect time to hunker down and let the cold wind blow.

JACK: Damn! It's cold out there. You would think just one weatherman could predict something like snow.

ANN: Snow? It's not snowing. It doesn't look like it's snowing?!

JACK: I don't care what it looks like. You go outside and there's cold wet shit coming down!

Excerpt from the play (A Matter of) Grace by Mary Miller

December 17th

The Miracle of Light

Every year it is customary to commemorate the miracle of Hanukkah for eight days by lighting candles on a menorah. It's the story of how one small bottle of oil, enough for only one day, was able miraculously to keep the lamp lit for eight days. It's a wonderful story of miracles, faith, hope, and light. Although the date of the celebration changes from year to year the miracle itself is constant.

A few minutes later, Fred walked out of the hotel with the unfolded map in his hand and the desk clerk following behind. As he walked to the car, the desk clerk continued to talk, pointing left, then right, and then left again twice. Fred smiled and nodded as he attempted to absorb the directions. He opened the car door and sat behind the wheel, next to Abigail, as the desk clerk leaned in the window and continued to tick off instructions. Fred simply smiled as the clerk gave him the complimentary pen and wished him good luck.

The car started on the second try. As they drove off, the clerk stood on the curb and waved good-bye. "Merry Christmas," he yelled. "Happy Hanukkah" he added making sure he'd covered all the holiday bases.

Excerpt from the book <u>A Christmas House</u> by Mary Miller

December 18th

Setting the stage ... for the holidays.

This is the time of year we change our stage to that of a winter wonderland. We bring trees inside. We hang stockings over the fireplace. We decorate everything in red and green. We even hang mistletoe from the ceiling and it gives us all an excuse to kiss a perfect stranger! See how easily your stage can change ... it's the holidays after all.

In the center of the room, the Christmas tree stood fully decorated with brightly-colored balls, red striped candy canes and icicles that glistened like silver. The girls had made the house a home ... a wonderful Christmas house decorated just like their home in Atlanta. Abigail swallowed hard. "Oh, my," she quietly said as her daughters sprang from their hiding places shouting, "MERRY CHRISTMAS."

Excerpt from the book A Christmas House by Mary Miller

December 19th

Re-writes

As with all great plays there will be re-writes. No script has ever been submitted to any production house that wasn't re-written. Your first draft is just that … your first draft. But once you have something down on paper, trust me, it's so much easier to make revisions. So don't be afraid to write your play … and don't be adverse to making changes. Theatre is a living breathing thing … just as life … there are do-overs and re-writes!

MATTIE: You're a good writer, Chandler. You should write.

Excerpt from the play <u>Virgin Tears</u> by Mary Miller

December 20th

Re-staging

No matter how hard you work and how much you try there will always be changes to your set. Some maybe natural disasters that can tear the entire thing down ... others won't be so drastic but can be just as devastating. When your child goes off to college or you lose a loved one, the cast of characters you have on your stage will change from time to time for better or worse. But that is the nature of drama. It's part of the story. It evolves and changes and keeps us on our toes.

CHANDLER: (CONT.) Will you tell Adele, good-bye? I don't want to risk another scene.

Excerpt from the play <u>Virgin Tears</u> by Mary Miller

December 21ˢᵗ

Re-spect

In the end always remember to respect yourself because no matter what play you play it all begins and ends with you. Think about it. Do you realize the longest relationship you will ever have with anyone is with yourself? Take a look in the mirror, a good long look. Love what you like, change what you don't. You are the great love of your life ... respect yourself.

WOMAN: Well, I couldn't go all the way in. Not without my uniform on and I wasn't about to wear my uniform to your Momma's grave. I got more respect for her than a J.C. Penney catalogue uniform.

CHILD: She didn't care what you got on?

WOMAN: I care.

Excerpt from the play <u>Take Proper Care</u> by Mary Miller

December 22nd

Believe

All great actors believe in the parts they play. They believe they are real and in the believing they become real. You have to believe what you say for it to have any lasting effect. The mind is a tricky thing. You can't fool it. You can't say you are great when you know you are not. But once you have found your strength focus on it, and that belief, in something positive, will be the linchpin in changing and believing what you say and think about yourself.

JANICE: They'll never believe that?

MIA: It's the truth!

Excerpt from the play <u>Waiting for Oprah</u> by Mary Miller

December 23rd

Holiday blues…

One thing I've noticed as I get older is that the holidays are often tainted with sorrow. As children the holidays are filled with wonder … as adults they can be filled with worry. If you find yourself succumbing to the holiday blues get up and move. It's hard to stay depressed when you are in motion. Go for a walk … around the room … around the block … around the mall … move it, move it, move it!

CLARICE: Well, what're you waiting for? Go on. Times a wasting! Move it!!

BERNICE: What do I look like, an Olympic Track Star! Give me a break. I'm going.

CLARICE: Move it! Move it! Move it!

BERNICE: I'm going. I'm going. I'm going.

Excerpt from the play Mulberry Lane by Mary Miller

December 24th

A Time For Giving

This is the time of year when giving comes naturally. The time of year we don't think twice about spending more than we should on the people we love. It's the time of year for forgiving and forgetting. It's a magical time of year when we sincerely wish everyone we meet a very Merry Christmas and a Happy New Year!!

BABS: Merry Christmas! Merry Christmas!!

Excerpt from the play <u>A Christmas House</u> by Mary Miller

December 25th

MERRY CHRISTMAS!

Go out and make it a great day. Regardless of your faith. Regardless of your beliefs. Regardless of your religion. Today is a day of celebration. Step off the stage your are on and embrace the joy. Go out and find a miracle ... they are all around you!!

"Oh, and Fred," Abigail added as she put her arm around his waist. "Next year, I really think we should start getting ready earlier," she snuggled in close, "... if we're going to invite everyone down." She looked at her family and kissed him on the cheek, "... don't you think?" Outside, the light from the morning sun shone on the house, and the large red brick home with white columns looked beautiful, and finished, and perfect.

Excerpt from the book <u>A Christmas House</u> by Mary Miller

December 26th

The Day After

The day after Christmas for most people is a let down. But for me it's a chance to relax. We made it through another year of gifts and high expectations. Today is a chance to reflect and remember what is really important and look around and give thanks for what we have ... no matter how little or how much. Ironically the day after Christmas is a day of thanksgiving!

BERNICE: Thank you!

Excerpt from the play <u>Mulberry Lane</u> by Mary Miller

December 27th

Rainy days.

When I was in LA the one thing that surprised me was the weather. It was beautiful ... everyday! At first I loved it and then it began to grate on my nerves. In New York, on beautiful days, I made it a practice to get out and make something of the day. In New York beautiful days, especially in the winter, are few and far between. But in LA, where every day is a beautiful day, that practice became exhausting! So what I learned in LA was to make time for a rainy day, whether it was raining or not.

ADELE: She was wrong about the weather. It's not going to rain.

MATTIE: No. It's a beautiful night.

Excerpt from the play <u>Virgin Tears</u> by Mary Miller

December 28th

The Pendulum Swings

When I was a child my father used to always compare life to a pendulum swinging. This was great when you were having a bad day ... but not so great when the day was good. But over all I've learned to take the good with the bad. Because nothing lasts forever and the pendulum always swings back.

ROBERT: (smiling) How long are you staying?

CHANDLER: (shrugging her shoulders) Until that statue cries.

ROBERT: Well then, that could be forever.

Excerpt from the play Waiting for Oprah by Mary Miller

December 29th

The Little Engine That Could

When I was a kid my favorite story was *The Little Engine That Could.* I loved the fact that no one thought the little engine could make it over the mountain except the little engine itself. "I think I can. I think I can." It's a mantra we all should adopt. How far can we go? Who knows? But if we think we can ... we can go a lot further then we ever expected. "I thought I could. I thought I could."

DORIE: My Daddy, he believed you should do something that frightens you at least once a year. Builds character. Strengthens moral fiber. You ought to try it sometime.

Excerpt from the play <u>Ferris Wheel</u> by Mary Miller

December 30th

The Role of a Lifetime.

Acting Healthy is not merely about putting on the costume, learning the lines, and getting into make up. Acting Healthy is about believing in the role so much it gets under your skin and into your heart. Acting Healthy is more than playing a character on stage; it's living that life every day. It's taking it so deep that when you look into a mirror you actually see a difference. You not only look thinner, you are thinner. You not only look happier, you are happier. You not only look healthier, you are healthier. You are whatever you imagine yourself to be. So, decide which play you want to live. Re-write the dialogue. Re-design the set. Re-cast yourself in the role of a lifetime.

MIA: I wonder, if you could live your life as a fictional character who would it be?

Excerpt from the play <u>Waiting for Oprah</u> by Mary Miller

December 31st

A New New Year's Resolution

This year why not make your New Year's resolution one to do whatever is best for you! I know it sounds selfish but often times I have found that if I take care of my needs first I'm better able to take care of others later. This year why not re-evaluate what you are doing. Ask yourself if it's good for you, your career, your family, and your life? These are big questions. Take your time. So often we let them slide by (without ever asking!) that by the time we do ... we think it's too late to change and give up without trying. I'm here to tell you it's never too late. Put your needs first ... that's a *new* New Year's Resolution that could be worth keeping all year!

WOMAN: I am taking what is rightfully mine.

MAN: Says who?

WOMAN: Says me.

Excerpt from the play Patterson's by Mary Miller

January 1st

HAPPY NEW YEAR!!

_____
_____
_____

(Fill in the blank … it's your story now!)

ABOUT THE AUTHOR

Award-winning author and playwright, Mary Miller was born and raised in Atlanta, GA, and graduated with honors from Westminster High Schools. She received her B.A. at Hollins University in Roanoke, VA, after having studied at the University of London in London, England, and Davidson College in Davidson, NC. She gained her theatrical experience from years of work in New York City, first as an actress and then as a playwright.

As an actress she appeared both on stage (Off-Off Broadway) as well as on television. For two years she worked on the daytime soap opera *All My Children*. Preferring writing to acting Mary turned her attention to plays. She made her New York debut as a playwright with the production of LIGHT BURGERS WALTZING THROUGH THE GARDEN WITH JOE. She went on to win the Dayton Playhouse Future Fest first with I WITNESS and then again with WAITING FOR OPRAH. After the publication of her short play FERRIS WHEEL in the anthology TAKE TEN by Vintage Books/Random House, her work began to receive international attention. Since then she has written a number of both full length and short plays, won over a dozen national playwriting awards and had her work produced throughout the United States and the world.

After living in New York City, Mary moved to St. Simons Island off the coast of Georgia, where she continues to write and see her work produced. On St. Simons Island, she became involved in radio and worked for WMOG hosting the "Open Mike" show, a live morning call-in program. From radio she moved into television working for WBSG-TV. There she wrote, produced, and served as anchor on the half-hour television series "Close-Up 21".

Having gained success as a playwright, Mary turned her hand to novels and has written A CHRISTMAS HOUSE and A MATTER OF GRACE.

Currently she is focusing her attention on a health and wellness program she created called ACTING HEALTHY. Acting Healthy is a new approach to wellness using tips and techniques she first learned as an actress and then embraced as a writer to help people play a bigger, happier, thinner, younger, healthier part in their own lives! Her book ACTING HEALTHY – DIRECTORS NOTES FOR A BETTER LIFE is a daily journal designed to give the reader the directions they need to live that better life … day after day.

www.actinghealthy.com

For more information about her books, plays, and wellness programs please visit her website.

www.marymillerwriter.com

Also by MARY MILLER

NOVELS:
A Christmas House
A Matter of Grace

PLAYS:
Full-Length Plays
I Witness
A Christmas House
Light Burgers Waltzing Through the Garden with Joe
Virgin Tears on Wyoming Avenue
(A Matter of) Grace
Waiting for Oprah

Short Plays & Ten-Minute Plays
Ferris Wheel
Mulberry Lane
Take Proper Care
"Next"
Patterson's
At 3:00 O'clock in the Morning